Plenty of Room for Biology

at the Bottom

An Introduction to Bionanotechnology

Second Edition

Plenty of Room for Biology

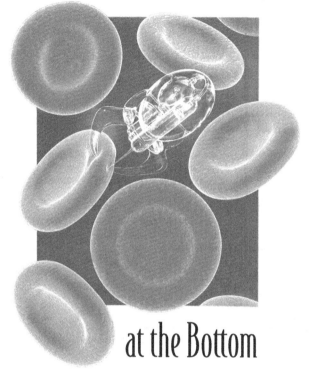

at the Bottom

An Introduction to Bionanotechnology

Second Edition

Ehud Gazit
Tel Aviv University, Israel

Anna Mitraki
University of Crete and IESL-FORTH, Greece

Imperial College Press

ICP

Published by

Imperial College Press
57 Shelton Street
Covent Garden
London WC2H 9HE

Distributed by

World Scientific Publishing Co. Pte. Ltd.
5 Toh Tuck Link, Singapore 596224
USA office: 27 Warren Street, Suite 401-402, Hackensack, NJ 07601
UK office: 57 Shelton Street, Covent Garden, London WC2H 9HE

Library of Congress Cataloging-in-Publication Data
Gazit, Ehud.
    Plenty of room for biology at the bottom : an introduction to bionanotechnology / by Ehud Gazit,
Tel Aviv University, Israel & Anna Mitraki,
University of Crete and Institute for Electronic Structure and Laser, Greece. -- Second edition.
    pages cm
    Includes bibliographical references and index.
    ISBN 978-1-84816-930-2 (hardcover : alk. paper)
    1. Biotechnology. 2. Biomimetic materials. 3. Biomolecules. 4. Nanotechnology.
5. Biomimetics. I. Mitraki, Anna. II. Title.
    QP514.2.G39 2013
    610.28--dc23
                                                        2012048470

British Library Cataloguing-in-Publication Data
A catalogue record for this book is available from the British Library.

Typeset by Stallion Press
Email: enquiries@stallionpress.com

Printed in Singapore

This book is dedicated to my family with love (E.G.)

To my two mentors, Professor Jeannine Yon-Kahn
of Université Paris-Sud, France and
Professor Jonathan King
of MIT, USA (A.M.)

Contents

Preface

This book represents a great challenge: It introduces the readers to the integration of two of the most important disciplines of the 21st century, biotechnology and nanotechnology. A special effort was made to expose readers from diverse backgrounds to the basic principles, techniques, applications, and great prospects at the intersection of these two key fields. All of this is done without assuming a strong background in either of the two subjects. We will discuss two related fields: "nanobiotechnology" which relates to the application nanotechnological principles and tools to biology, but also "bionanotechnology" which concerns the use of biological principles such as recognition and assembly for nanotechnological applications.

While the 20th century was the century of physics, electronics, and communication, the years to come are considered to be mainly dominated by the biological revolution that already started in the second half of the 20th century as well as nanotechnology, a new and exciting front that deals with minuscule nanometer-scaled assemblies and devices. Traditionally, miniaturization was a process in which devices became smaller and smaller by continuous improvement of existing techniques. Yet, we rapidly approach the limits of miniaturization using the conventional top-down fabrication tools. One of the key futuristic ways of making tiny machines will be to scale them up from the molecular level. For that purpose, many lessons could be learned about the arrangement of nano-scale machines as occurs in each and every biological system. The living cell is actually the only place in which genuine functional molecular machines, as often described in futuristic presentations of nanotechnology, could actually be found. Molecular motors, ultrasensitive nano-scale sensors, DNA replication machines, protein synthesis machines, and many other miniature devices exist even in the very simple early prebacterial cells that evolved more than three billion years ago. When we climb higher up the evolution tree, the nano-machines of course become more sophisticated and powerful. Yet, only billions of years after life emerged, we are beginning to utilize the concepts of recognition and assembly that lead to the formation of nano-scale machines for our technological needs. On the other hand many principles and applications of nano-technology that were developed for non-biological systems could be very useful for immediate biological applications such as advanced sensors and molecular scaffolds for tissue engineering as well as long-term prospects such as *in situ* modifications at the protein and DNA levels.

While the fields of nanobiotechnology and bionanotechnology are very new their prospects are immense. The marriage between biotechnology and nanotechnology could lead to a dramatic advancement in the medical sciences. It may well be a place in which many of the current diseases and human disorders will be eradicated. In a reasonable time-scale, cancer and AIDS may be regarded in the same way that polio and tuberculosis are being considered now. Genetic defects could be identified and corrected even before birth. Nano-scale robots that may be inserted into our body could perform very complicated surgical tasks such as a brain surgery. Nano-machines may even be able to solve problems on the cellular level. Manipulation of the genetic information inside the body in real-time is only one example.

The principles of biological recognition could also serve as the basis for applications that seem to be very far from living systems as we identify them. One of the most obvious directions in the field of nanotechnology will be molecular electronics. The use of the tools of molecular recognition between biomolecules and their ability to self-assemble into elaborated structures could actually serve as an excellent model system for the 21st century nano-engineers. This course of study will link us directly to the one of the most important areas of research and development of the second half of the 20th century, the silicon-based microelectronics. Biology-based nanotechnology may facilitate our ability to overcome many of the limitations of the silicon-based world, as we know them today. The field of electronics could be transformed to have complete new and exciting prospects when electronic devices will be made by nano-machines and be governed by molecular self-assembly principles. The world after this bionanotechnologic revolution may be a place where the molecular mechanism of thinking and reasoning will be understood and truly artificial intelligence machines could be manufactured.

It should always be remembered that the new era of nanobiotechnology and bionanotechnology may also lead to a situation in which there will be a very fine line between prosperity and devastation. The role of the scientists and technologists in the years to come will be to ensure the proper usage of these hardly imaginable abilities. We must make sure this revolution will be used for the benefit of mankind and not for its destruction. As those tools are so powerful, their misuse may actually lead to grave consequences.

E. Gazit

It was a great pleasure to join in the updating of the second edition of this book and I hope it will be a useful resource for colleagues and students from a variety of disciplines.

In updating this book, care was taken to preserve the original spirit of the book as much as possible, i.e. to introduce readers from diverse backgrounds to the intersection of biotechnology and nanotechnology without assuming any prior knowledge. We have therefore tried to convey the essence of key developments made since the first edition of the book without becoming too extensive or specific. Key scientific discoveries are included, such as the discovery of graphene and the complete structure of the ribosome, which have recently won Nobel prizes (Chapters 2 and 3). The sections on nanoscale bioassemblies (Chapter 3) are expanded to include recent structural and biological information, for example on amyloid-type assemblies. Care is taken to introduce the readers to recent web tools that visualization of biological structures, such as Proteopedia, the three-dimensional interactive encyclopedia created by scientists in 2009. Chapter 6 on self-assembly of biological and bio-inspired materials is expanded to include more building blocks. The effervescence of recent literature on biological templates for the production of inorganic composite materials is reflected in the enlarged Chapter 7, which focuses on application of biological assemblies in nanotechnology. In Chapter 8, which focuses on medical and other applications of bionanotechnology, advances concerning the use of biological nanotubes in sensing, biological detection, and integration in devices are underlined. Finally, in Chapter 9, future prospects on tissue engineering, and the convergence of "bottom-up" and "top-down" fabrication strategies are briefly discussed.

I would like to thank Dr. Panagiotis Argitis of Demokritos, Athens, for his useful input, especially concerning the current limits of lithography in Chapter 1.

A. Mitraki

Chapter 1

Introduction: Nanobiotechnology and Bionanotechnology

The convergence of the scientific disciplines of biotechnology and nanotechnology is a relatively recent one. Yet, the combination of these highly important areas of research has already resulted in remarkable achievements. This chapter will provide basic background on classical and modern biotechnology and its interface with nanotechnology, a much less mature scientific discipline. Throughout this book we will use the term "nanobiotechnology" to describe the applications of nanotechnology techniques for the development and improvement of biotechnological process and products. This includes the use of fabrication and manipulation techniques at the nano-scale to form more sensitive and accurate diagnosis methods such as a "lab-on-a-chip", point-of-care (POC) diagnostics, and real-time nano-sensors. This also includes the use of matrices of nano-scale order for the controlled release of drugs as well as tissue engineering and regeneration. Later on in the book, we will describe more advanced futuristic directions such as the development of devices that allow manipulations at the nano-scale ("nano-robots") to perform medical procedures in patients or nano-machines that could serve as artificial alternatives to functional biological organs.

The term "bionanotechnology" will be employed to describe the use of biological building blocks and the utilization of biological specificity and activity for the development of modern technology at the nano-scale. Such bionanotechnology practice is obviously not limited to biological applications but have much wider scope. For instance, futuristic applications of bionanotechnology could include the use of DNA oligomers, peptide nanotubes, or protein fibrils for the fabrication of metal nanowires, interconnects or other physical elements at the nano-scale, that could be used in molecular electronics and nano-electromechanical applications and devices (Braun *et al.*, 1998; de la Rica *et al.*, 2008; Patolsky *et al.*, 2004a; Patolsky *et al.*, 2004b; Reches and Gazit, 2003; Smith *et al.*, 2011; Zhang, 2003).

1.1. Classical Biotechnology: Industrial Production Using Biological Systems

Biotechnology is a well-established scientific discipline. The practice of classical biotechnology, defined by the American Heritage Dictionary as "The use of microorganisms, such as bacteria or yeasts, or biological substances, such as enzymes, to perform specific industrial or manufacturing processes", goes back to the first half of the 20th century (Figure 1.1). The large-scale industrial application of biological processes, such as the production of acetone by the fermentation of starch with the bacterium *Clostridium acetobutylicum*, was already performed in 1916. The industrial production of penicillin antibiotics from *Penicillium notatum* bacteria for practical medical use was already achieved in the early 1940s.

Other scholars attribute the use of biotechnology practice to a much earlier era as a variety of food products, such as wine, beer, cheese, and bread had already been produced with the help of yeasts and bacteria for a few thousand years, from the early days of civilization (Figure 1.1).

Figure 1.1:   Milestones in the development of modern biotechnology into bionanotechnology. Production of bread, wine, and yogurt was practiced thousands of years before the commercial production of acetone, antibiotics, and biological drugs.

1.2. Modern Biotechnology: From Industrial Processes to Novel Therapeutics

Over the years, the practical definition of biotechnology became much more vague. Much of the activity of the modern biotechnology practice, both in the academic settings as well as the industrial ones, developed into applied biological sciences rather than a well-defined scientific discipline. The activity that is described as "biotechnology" ranges from the production of biomolecules (e.g. functional proteins or antibodies) to serve as drugs to the development of novel diagnostic tools that are based on the interaction of specific biomolecules (such as antibody-antigen interactions as in immunodiagnostic kits or complementary nucleic acid interactions as in DNA-array microchips). The somewhat practical distinction between the pharmaceutical industry and the modern biotechnology industry is the production of large biomolecules such as functional proteins and antibodies by the latter as compared to small molecule drugs by the former.

For example, the first product of the largest biotechnology company, *Amgen*, is an industrially produced naturally occurring protein denoted erythropoietin (commercial name: EPOGEN®) that stimulates the production of red blood cells. This product was approved for human use in 1989 by the Food and Drug Administration (FDA) and represents one of the very first modern biotechnology products. Other biotechnology products include recombinant human insulin, human interferon, human and bovine growth hormones, and therapeutic antibodies. The production of therapeutic antibodies is especially intriguing and represents a relatively new area of research. These therapeutic agents utilize the notable affinity and selectivity of antibodies (as described in Chapter 4) to block harmful biological processes by a directed and remarkably specific manner. A recent example is the humanized recombinant monoclonal antibody that binds to and inhibits the biochemical activity of the vascular endothelial growth factor (commercial name: AVASTIN™). This antibody-based treatment significantly increases the survival rates of patients with metastatic carcinoma of the colon that is incurable by conventional chemotherapy. Another major biotechnological product that was mentioned above is human interferon, a protein that has a central role in the response of the human body to viral infection, and human growth hormone, a key regulator of normal growth of children and adolescents.

Many more proteins are now been developed for their use as potential drugs. One of the limiting factors for a much more common use of protein and peptide drugs is their unavailability in oral formulation. Unlike small molecule drugs, which are commonly administered in the form of tablets or syrup, protein and peptide drugs are usually degraded during their passage in the digestive track. Therefore, the administration of the protein and peptide drugs as mentioned above is limited to injections that cannot easily be performed by the patients outside of medical institutions. Another application of peptide and protein drugs is topical, which again is very limited in its therapeutic scope. Actually, in this case nanotechnology can provide a very helpful and important solution. For example, arrays of hundreds or thousands of tiny nano-syringes are used for dermal application of biomolecular agents without any associated pain. Other applications including various nano-carriers are being studied for their ability to safely transfer drugs throughout most of the digestive track, but release them at the intestines. Nano-carriers are also being studied for their ability to allow the transfer of protein and peptide drugs through the blood–brain barrier (BBB) to treat diseases such as brain tumors and various neuro-degenerative disorders. The nano-carriers themselves can be formed by the self-assembly of biomaterials (such as peptide nano-spheres) but can also be composed of nonbiological materials. At any rate, this is an example for the way in which nanotechnology can help biotechnology to reach much wider use.

1.3. Modern Biotechnology: Immunological, Enzymatic, and Nucleic Acid-Based Technology

The diagnostic aspect of biotechnology principally consists of the detection and quantification of biological materials using biochemical techniques such as immunological recognition assays, enzymatic reactions, and DNA- or RNA-based technology. As will be discussed in this book, the use of nano-scale assemblies and fabrication may help to significantly improve the sensitivity, as well as the specificity, of the diagnosis process.

Diagnostic immunoassays include products such as the home pregnancy test kits that contain antibodies that detect minute traces of the human chorionic gonadotropin (hCG) hormone (Cole, 1997). Other products include diagnostic kits for the determination of human immuno-deficiency virus (HIV) or hepatitis virus infections. In all these cases a specific high affinity and specificity molecular recognition process facilitates the diagnosis process. The chemical basis for this recognition, specificity, and affinity will be further elaborated in this book. Understanding and miniaturization of the detectors and molecular markers of the recognition process will lead to better utilization of these interactions for various diagnostic applications. The increased sensitivity of such devices will result in the need for much lower volumes of blood to determine specific key biological parameters such as the glucose levels (Figure 1.2). Actually this lower amount of blood, which could be reduced from micro-liters to nano-liters, can be extracted by the nano-syringes mentioned above that will significantly reduce the discomfort associated with the collection of blood samples for glucose levels determination. A more futuristic instrument may include a nano-device that measures the glucose levels using electrochemical reaction and nano-electrodes on a chip that are connected to a controlled delivery system that releases insulin according to a programmed profile. Such a

Figure 1.2: Detection of glucose level is based on the combination of enzymatic reaction and electrochemical detection. Hydrogen peroxide is being formed upon the oxidation of glucose by the glucose oxidase (GOX) enzyme. The level of the redox reaction is being determined electrochemically. In principle, the reaction can be performed on a nano-scale as the size of the enzyme is less than 10 nm.

nano-device will be able to mimic some of the functions of the pancreas for acute type I and chronic type II diabetes patients.

The diagnostic use of enzymatic reactions includes common instruments such as home glucometers that utilize the catalytic reaction of the glucose oxidase enzyme with glucose to produce gluconic acid and hydrogen peroxide (Jaffari and Turner, 1995). The latter chemical product is being electrochemically determined and converted into a digital output (Figure 1.2). This is indeed one of the key examples of the merging between biotechnology and electronics to produce a hybrid enzyme–electronic interface. Miniaturization of such and other enzyme-based detectors is one of the envisioned nanobiotechnological devices (Jaremko and Rorstad, 1998).

DNA-based technology includes the polymerase chain reaction (PCR) process that is being extensively used in forensic science to clearly determine the source of biological samples. Another technique that utilizes the specificity of nucleic acids interaction is the DNA microarray chip technology. This technology allows following the expression pattern of thousands or even tens of thousands of genes simultaneously. The DNA-array techniques are not only invaluable to basic medical studies but they also pave the way for future personal medicine. Also, these applications can be significantly advanced by the use of nanotechnology, for example by performing the reactions at very small volume using "lab-on-a-chip" settings. This should allow much smaller amounts of biological samples for the application of the nucleic acid based techniques. Such an increase in sensitivity should be especially helpful in forensic science and in the early detection of pathological processes such as early phase of malignant transformation. Other very important applications may include environmental monitoring and homeland security detection of biological and chemical agents.

1.4. The Interface Between Nanotechnology and Biotechnology: Bionanotechnology

As mentioned above, nanotechnology is a relatively young scientific discipline. Chapter 2 provides some of the basic themes and principles of nanotechnology that are mainly directed at readers with a background in the biological sciences. As a basic introduction, nanotechnology could be described as technological applications using systems and devices with orders at the nanometer scale (as most of the readers are aware, one nanometer equals one-thousandth of a micrometer or one-millionth of a millimeter — 1/1,000,000,000 meter). The study of nanotechnology includes molecular systems, molecular assemblies (such as quantum dots), tubular and spherical nanostructures, and well-organized self-assembled devices and machines. All these are considered to be part of the "bottom-up" approach in which simple components at the nanometric scale join together to form complex machines, devices, or instruments by spontaneous processes that involve molecular recognition and self-assembly events.

Biology and biological recognition should have great importance in these directions of molecular recognition and self-assembly. Biomolecules and biological complexes are naturally occurring building blocks, recognition modules, and even machines (such as the ribosome, the complex protein assembly line, or molecular motors). Even more complex structures such as plant and animal viruses or bacteriophages (viruses that attack bacteria) could be formed by association at the nano-scale. Biological recognition, such as the one attained by specific antibodies (see Chapter 4), can specifically direct the "bottom-up" assembly. By the utilization of the high specificity and the spontaneity of biological association processes, biological assemblies can serve as a "smart scaffold" for the self-association of complex organic and inorganic nano-machines and nano-devices.

Other directions are the "top-down" approaches, which consist of either continuous improvement of common ultraviolet (UV) lithographic processes or the use of more elaborate lithographic technologies such as electron-beam (E-beam) lithography or focused ion beam (FIB) lithography. As of 2011, industrial scale lithography, used in the field of microelectronics, already reached a 22 nm resolution by the use of 193 nm deep ultraviolet photolithography. Electromagnetic radiation of shorter wavelength was demonstrated to be useful at even better resolution. Furthermore, the use of a beam of electrons or ions instead of photons allows the fabrication of objects at even higher resolution (as low as few nm).

There is no doubt that these techniques, either the "bottom-up" or "top-down", will revolutionize the field of biotechnology. The above-mentioned biotechnological techniques and procedures and many others could extensively benefit from their interfacing with modern nanotechnology techniques. This may be merely the miniaturization that will result in much simpler procedures that will require significantly smaller volumes of biological samples and will make the medical procedures much simpler and more pleasant to the patient. Yet, it could lead to the assembly of sophisticated machines at the nano-scale that do not only measure but also perform various tasks that are based on these measurements. Moreover, the interface of biotechnology and nanotechnology can offer the attainment of sensitivities that are orders of magnitudes higher than current techniques. The ability to determine the presence of the very first cancerous cell in the body or the monitoring of minute amounts of pollutants or volatile explosives will dramatically revolutionize the medical practice as well as homeland security and environmental monitoring.

1.5. Supramolecular (Bio)Chemistry: The Theoretical Basis for Self-Assembly

Supramolecular chemistry consists of the study of the structure and function of the entities formed by association of two or more chemical species by noncovalent interactions. These types of supramolecular structures are actually types of "supermolecules" that are distinct from regular molecules that are being formed by continuous chemical covalent bonding between atoms. To distinguish between supramolecular structures and covalent chemical structures, we will usually use the term "assemblies" to describe the noncovalent structures.

The foundations of this field of science were laid down only a few decades ago. The founding fathers are considered to be Donald J. Cram, Jean-Marie Lehn, and Charles J. Pedersen who were awarded the Nobel Prize in Chemistry in 1987. The citation of the prize reads "for their development and use of molecules with structure-specific interactions of high selectivity". According to one definition suggested by Lehn: "supramolecular chemistry is chemistry beyond the molecule". It should be noted that the term "supermolecules" was already coined in the 1930s (Pfeffer, 1927), yet the exact description of the complex chemical interactions that lead to the formation of these ordered structures was yet to be described decades later.

It is also worth noting that while this notion of supramolecular assemblies is relatively new, many biological entities can be considered as supramolecular assemblies. These can be as simple as functional dimers (e.g., Fos–Jun transcription factor) and as complex as molecular nanomachines such as the ribosome or molecular motors. Taken together, biology can be considered as a most advanced playground of supramolecular chemistry as complex biology functions are being achieved through the formation of complex molecular structures by noncovalent interactions (Aizenberg *et al.*, 2005). Throughout this book we will consider self-assembly and molecular-recognition (see below) as central themes in bionanotechnology and nanobiotechnology.

These processes in which large ordered assemblies are being formed by noncovalent association of simpler building blocks are the essence of "bottom-up" design. In this approach simple building blocks are joined together to form supermolecules or assemblies that have a distinct morphology and often also specific function or unique physicochemical properties.

1.6. The Next Steps for Self-Association at the Nano-Scale

The formation of ordered structures by self-association at the nano-scale is just the first step toward the formation of ordered molecular structures. The next steps involve the formation of heterocomponent assemblies, such as observed with the biomolecular assemblies and machines described above. The formation of such structures should be based on the combination of recognition modules that are evolving from geometrical complementary (Figure 1.3) but also on chemical recognition. Elements such as aromatic moieties that combine both properties are especially attractive elements in the self-association design schemes. This is due to the geometrically restricted nature of these interactions on the one hand, and to the specific entropic and enthalpic chemical interaction on the other hand. It has already been shown that well ordered structures, such as peptide nanotubes, could self-assemble by the facilitation of such interactions (e.g., Reches and Gazit, 2003).

As will be discussed in Chapter 4, it was already demonstrated that many complex structures could be formed by the self-association of

Figure 1.3: Self-assembly of molecules into ordered noncovalent structures at the nano-scale. In the current example complementary geometry is directing the association. Yet, other factors such as chemical complementarity may facilitate such multicomponent association.

biomolecules. The pioneering work by Nadrian Seeman and coworkers had demonstrated the ability of partially complementary DNA strands, which form molecular junctions, to self-assemble into two-dimensional nanowires and three-dimensional nanocubes (Seeman, 1990; 2005; 2010). Other researchers had demonstrated the ability of peptide molecules to self-assemble into tubes, spheres, plates, tapes, and hydrogels with nano-scale order (Aggeli *et al.*, 1997; Altman *et al.*, 2000; Bong *et al.*, 2001; Banerjee *et al.*, 2003; Ghadiri *et al.*, 1993, 1994; Silva *et al.*, 2004). Such nano-scale peptide assemblies were already proven to have potential in diverse fields such as tissue engineering and regeneration (Hauser and Zhang, 2010; Holmes *et al.*, 2000; Silva *et al.*, 2004), the design of novel antibacterial agents that form nanochannels (Ghadiri *et al.*, 1994), and the fabrication of metallic nanowires (Reches and Gazit, 2003).

1.7. Biology in Nanotechnology and Nano-Sciences in Biotechnology

As already mentioned above, the practice of biology or biotechnology at the nano-scale could be divided into two main categories (Figure 1.4). The first one is the technological applications of self-assembled nano-scale ordered biomolecular in various fields. These disciplines may not have any biological relevance *per se*. The role of biology in these cases is mainly based on its remarkable specificity and diversity and its ability to facilitate the formation of very complex nanostructures by relatively simple building

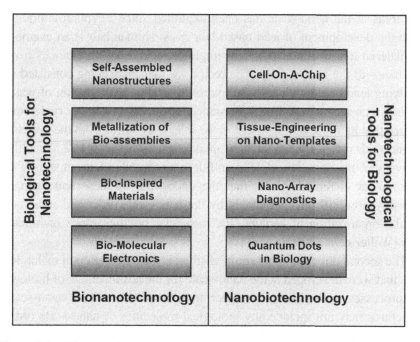

Figure 1.4: Bionanotechnology as the use of biological assemblies for various applications that may not be directionally associated with biology. Nanobiotechnology is the use of nano-science for specific biological applications.

blocks. We would refer to this direction as bionanotechnology, the application of biology and biomolecules into technological applications at the nano-scale. These directions will be extensively described in this book. Yet, as an introduction, we would like to mention the use of biomolecules (such as DNA and proteins) for the fabrication of metallic structures at the nano-scale (Patolsky *et al.*, 2004a; Reches and Gazit, 2003). Such structures can serve in future computers or other devices that may have no direct association with biology. Yet, the biology may provide tools that are not currently available by any other means. This was illustrated by the practice of molecular lithography in which protein molecules of few nano-meters served as a resist for the fabrication of gold wires on DNA molecules (Keren *et al.*, 2002 — see Chapter 7). Other directions may include the formation of novel materials of unique rigidity, surface chemistry, or other physicochemical properties that may prove useful in the automobile or space industries or simply in consumer goods. It is worth noticing that the ability of biological molecules to template the formation of inorganic materials at the nano-scale has been exploited since Egyptian antiquity, with the development of lead-based hair dyes. Human hair is an example of material that is organized from simple molecular building blocks from the nano- to the macro-scale. The recipe for hair blackening consisted in applying lead oxide with calcium hydroxide and a small amount of water to form a paste. An experiment reproduced in a modern laboratory demonstrated that hair blackening is due to the release of sulfur from the cysteine amino acids in hair (due to the very alkaline environment, pH 12.5) and the subsequent precipitation of lead sulfide nanocrystals of average size of 5nm. What is remarkable is that the deposition of these nanocrystals (roughly every 10 nm) is dictated by the nano-scale order and supramolecular organization of keratins, the molecular building block of human hair (Walter *et al.*, 2006).

The second direction that is quite distinct is the application of technologies that were developed at the nano-scale for the advancement of biological processes, such as tissue engineering or diagnostics. These nano-scale structures may not include any biological molecules of nano-scale order as they could completely utilize silicon-based structures (such as in the case of a "lab-on-a-chip") or carbon nanostructures (such as in the case of tissue engineering on carbon nanotube-based substrates). Such an application could actually revolutionize the field of biotechnology by allowing the early diagnosis of disease, the online monitoring of therapeutic procedures, and the formation of tissue in the test tubes.

It is worth mentioning that the actual use of the terms "nanobiotechnology" or "bionanotechnology" is quite a recent one. According to the *MedLine* database, the term "nanobiotechnology" appears first in 2000, while the first hit for "bionanotechnology" is only in 2004. "Nanobiotechnology" is notably more than four times more common that "bionanotechnology". Yet, in many of the cases the use of the latter term would have been much more appropriate.

1.8. The Combination of Bionanotechnology and Nanobiotechnology

In spite of the distinction between bionanotechnology and nanobiotechnology, it should be stressed for future applications, especially complex ones, that both fields could be merged. For example, in the field of tissue engineering, self-assembled biomolecular structures could serve as a three-dimensional template for the formation of complex organs in the test tube. In these applications, the biomolecules serve exactly as the nano-carbon structures as mentioned above. Nevertheless, the biomolecular nano-scaffold may provide unique advantages such as biocompatibility and the ability of decoration with biological signaling motifs. Self-assembling peptides that form hydrogels mimicking the extracellular matrix can incorporate growth factors and have been recently designed to display cell-binding motifs and/or to incorporate protease sites for remodeling. Such multifunctional artificial matrices are promising materials in three-dimensional cell culture and regenerative medicine in the near future (Collier *et al.*, 2010). In the field of nano-bio-diagnostics, peptide nanotubes could serve as nano-scale elements for the improvement of the sensitivity of signals and specificity. Here again the biomolecular nano-scale assemblies serve in principle just as the carbon or inorganic nanostructures. Yet, the biological nanotubes have many advantages as they provide a unique anchor for the conjugation of signal-enhancing entities like enzymes or antibodies. To illustrate a recent example, a peptide-nanotube-based, label-free sensor for the detection of viruses was developed by positioning a peptide nanotube coated with antivirus antibodies between an electrode gap. The binding event of virus to the antibody could be detected by the capacitance change (de La Rica *et al.*, 2011). Ultimately, one could imagine that peptide nanotubes could serve both as recognition elements and sensing elements in a sensor.

1.9. Nanobionics and Bio-Inspired Nanotechnology

The final introduction to the field of nanobiology (we will use this term to describe both bionanotechnology and nanobiotechnology) should also include bionics and bio-inspired technology. Bionics, which stems from bi(o)- + (electr)onics, could be described as the application of biological principles and mechanisms to the design and fabrication of engineering systems. Although the term "bionic" was coined only in the late 1950s by the US Air Force, these principles were already explored many years before. One the earliest examples and most significant examples are the studies of Leonardo da Vinci at the end of the 15th century (Figure 1.5). His famous suggestions for the principles of a helicopter were based on his studies and extensive observation of the flight of birds. Other bionic applications include the use of the nose of the dolphin as a model for a

Figure 1.5: The drawing of a flying machine, based on natural principles of the flying mechanism of birds, made by Leonardo da Vinci at the end of the 15th century.

pear-shaped bow protuberance of ships or self-cleaning surfaces that are based on the surface properties of lotus leaves. It should be stressed that the aim of bionics is not merely to copy nature but rather to understand its principles and use them as a stimulus and motivation for innovations. Thus, bio-inspired technology may be a more suitable name to describe this activity.

As most bionics is based on the formation of macroscopic objects and machines, it could also include nano-scale machines. It is expected that in years to come, the same mimicking as was performed in the macroscopic world will also be applied to the microscopic and nanoscopic world. This includes simple applications such as self-cleaning surfaces at the nano-scale but could be explored for the formation of much more complex structures such as molecular motors or even molecular machines.

Chapter 2

A Brief Introduction to Nanotechnology

Nanotechnology, in its broadest definition, is related to the study and technological applications of materials and assemblies at the nanometric scale. The common symbol for nanometer is "nm" (as a reminder, one nm is one-billionth of a meter — about the size of a small molecule that consists of few atoms). The prefix *nano* originated from the Greek word *nanos*, which literally means "dwarf". Traditionally nanotechnology was considered to be related to the study of objects smaller than 100 nm. However, for the discussion of nanobiotechnology and bionanotechnology at large, we will also discuss assemblies at the 100–500 nm range (e.g., small unilamellar lipid vesicles or liposomes that are being used for drug delivery applications). In this chapter we will give a brief summary of the history and current trends in nanotechnology research and applications without the assumption of any previous knowledge. This is done in order to give the appropriate introduction for readers with biological or other nonphysical background. While the introduction is quite short, it should allow for the understanding of the basics of biological branches of nanotechnology, nanobiotechnology or bionanotechnology.

2.1. The Emergence of Nanotechnology: "There's Plenty of Room at the Bottom"

Most scholars attribute the inauguration of modern nanotechnology to a very famous talk given by Prof. Richard P. Feynman on December 29th, 1959, at the annual meeting of the American Physical Society that was held at the California Institute of Technology. The legendary address, entitled *There's Plenty of Room at the Bottom. An Invitation to Enter a New Field of Physics* (the full transcript of the talk is provided in Appendix

A of this book), provided the first methodical introduction for the establishment of a new field of molecular manipulation. Feynman, a true maverick and one of the leading physicists of the 20th century who was awarded the 1965 Nobel Prize in Physics for his seminal work on quantum electrodynamics, suggested quite bluntly in his talk that it should be possible to manipulate molecules and atoms directly. Although he did not mention the term nanotechnology — his original statement was "What I want to talk about is the problem of manipulating and controlling things on a small scale" — he was genuinely the first person to define the uniqueness and the enormous potential of studies at the nanometric scale. He clearly stated that the principles of physics do not deny the possibility of manipulating things atom by atom. In his exciting and stimulating address Feynman discussed many issues ranging from data storage and fast computers to lubrication and evaporation at very small scales.

The relevance of Feynman's talk, almost half a century after it was delivered, is quite astonishing and reflects the vision and imagination of this great scientist. Many of the ideas that were raised in this classic public address are very relevant in our current time and even for future endeavors in nanotechnology. In fact, some of the challenges that were put forward tens of years ago, such as the fabrication of nano-scale motors, have not yet been achieved.

While Feynman is best known for his seminal contribution to modern physics, a very interesting point relates to his great interest in and affection towards the study of biology. He rejects the patronizing attitude of some of the physicists in the 1950s towards biologists — "I don't know any field where they are making more rapid progress than they are in biology today" — and suggests that what would eventually be termed as nanotechnology has both a lot to learn from biology as well as providing new and indispensable experimental tools for the biologists.

It will indeed take many years before biology will be integrated into the field of nanotechnology although, as was already mentioned and will be discussed below, biology is the only realm in which a handful of genuine nano-machines exist even in the simplest bacteria. Molecular nano-motors that we expect to be fabricated by advanced nanotechnology techniques are being produced by very primitive bacteria to serve as flagella and other swimming devices.

2.2. Coining the Term "Nanotechnology" and the Emergence of the Nanotechnology Concept

The actual coining of the term *"nanotechnology"* is attributed to Norio Taniguchi from Tokyo Science University, who first mentioned it in 1974. His definition for nanotechnology, which is still relevant in the 21st century, was: "'Nano-technology' mainly consists of the processing of separation, consolidation, and deformation of materials by one atom or one molecule" (Taniguchi, 1974).

Much of the later driving force to make nanotechnology a major scientific field should be credited to K. Eric Drexler (Drexler, 1981; 1986; 1992). In 1981 he had already published an article in the *Proceedings of the US National Academy of Science* in which he described how biological protein assemblies can serve as functional units such as motors, cables, and pumps at the nano-scale (Drexler, 1981). In this article Drexler very nicely stated that the components that are available in every living cell are comparable to components used for mechanical engineering. Drexler's 1986 book entitled *Engines of Creation: The Coming Era of Nanotechnology* is a true milestone and a pivotal reference for the field on nanotechnology. This book is freely available on the Internet (see Drexler, 1986 for website address) and readers are highly encouraged to download it. A later, more technical yet excellent description of the foundations of nanotechnology and its potential uses can be found in Drexler's 1992 book *Nanosystems: Molecular Machinery, Manufacturing, and Computation.*

2.3. Manipulating Molecules: The Scanning Probe Microscopes

In his talk Feynman envisioned the ability to make smaller and smaller tools by a sequential miniaturization of machine shop tools — making tools that are one-tenth the scale of the current tools, then using these tools to make new set of tools that are one-hundredth scale of the common tools, and so on and so forth until the ability to manipulate atoms and molecules is achieved.

It took some years until such tools became available. Yet these tools came from quite a different origin. The major milestone was the invention of the scanning tunneling microscope (STM) by Gerd Binnig and Heinrich Rohrer at IBM's Zurich Research Labs (Binnig *et al.*, 1982), who won the

1986 Nobel Prize in Physics for this achievement. This was followed five years later by the invention of the atomic force microscope (AFM). These microscopes are quite different from any other microscope, either light or electron microscopes. Unlike conventional microscopes in which a beam of photons or electrons are used for the construction of images that are based on optical principles using optical or electromagnetic lenses, the STM and AFM microscopes are based on very fine scanning of the sample surface using an ultrafine tip. The image that is achieved is based either on the electrical tunneling properties of the matter (in the case of STM) or the topographical properties of the sample (in the case of AFM). The generic name for this type of microscope is known as a scanning probe microscope (SPM). The tip, or probe, scans over the surface of the sample and measures a tunneling current in the case of STM or the physical topography of the surface in the case of AFM (Figure 2.1). Older readers may think about the scanning of the tip as the diamond stylus that rides along in the groove of a vinyl record played on an old gramophone.

In principle, the specifications of the scanning probe machinery allow us to reach a single atom resolution and indeed the atomic organization of metallic substrates. In the case of biological samples, STMs generally cannot be used as conductivity of the sample is required for tunneling current, yet most of the biological molecules are insulators. Similarly, in the case of AFMs, atomic resolution could not be reached with biological

Figure 2.1: The principle of action of the AFM. A very fine tip travels over the surface of the sample. The topographic properties of the scanned surface affect the reflection of the laser light from the cantilever. The changes in the reflection are translated into a three-dimensional map of the scanned surface.

samples due to the soft nature and stickiness of the biological samples that result in interaction with the tip and stretching of the sample in the low nanometric scale. A significant improvement in the study of biological and other "soft materials" came with the introduction of tapping-mode AFM. In this mode, the probe oscillates at a resonant frequency and at amplitude setpoint while scanning across the surface of a sample. In that way, the amplitude of the oscillation of the probe is changed in relation to the topography of the surface of the sample and thus it allows the reconstruction a topographic image.

The first vivid demonstration of the ability to manipulate atoms at the nano-scale was the ability to spell "IBM" using 35 xenon atoms on a nickel surface, using a STM to move the atoms into their position (Figure 2.2). This demonstration by the IBM Fellows was later followed by the construction of the famous "quantum corrals" in which iron atoms are positioned in circular patterns. These atomic constructions are made by bringing the STM tip very close to the atoms in a way that the weak interatomic and

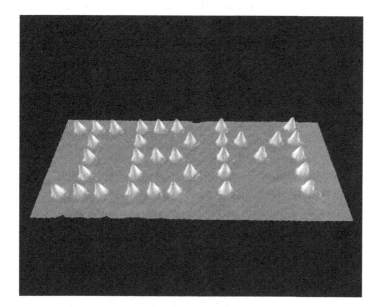

Figure 2.2: Spelling of "IBM" using 35 xenon atoms on a nickel surface. Courtesy of Dr. Donald Eigler. Reproduced by permission from Macmillan Publishers Ltd. [*Nature*], Eigler, D. M. and Schweizer, E. K. (1990) Positioning single atoms with a scanning tunneling microscope. *Nature* **344**, 524–526. Copyright 1990. Image originally created by IBM Corporation.

chemical forces between the tip and an individual atom move the atom to the desired position.

Scanning probe microscopy was later used for extended molecular organization purposes. The dip-pen nanolithography (DPN) technique that was developed by Chad A. Mirkin and coworkers uses AFM to introduce patterned molecules into surfaces (K.-B. Lee *et al.*, 2002; 2003). In this technique, the AFM tip is used to deliver molecules to a surface via a solvent meniscus, which naturally forms at the end of the tip in ambient atmosphere. The molecules are used as "ink" while the AFM tip is being used as a "pen". This technique is very useful for the patterning of biological molecules at a resolution that is better than 50 nm.

2.4. Carbon Fullerene: A New Form of Carbon

Much of the current everyday chemistry is based on the use of organic compounds, which means molecules that are based on carbon as a key building block. Almost one-fifth of the weight of the human body is carbon, which is more than any other element except oxygen. Not only are most biological entities such as proteins, nucleic acids, and lipids organic compounds but much of the common industrial products such as nylon, plastic, Teflon, etc. are made of carbon as a key constituent. Also new materials including hyper-strong but lightweight materials such as KEVLAR® are based on organic entities such as aromatic amides. The use of aromatic moieties for fibril formation will be described later in the book. Organic chemistry in general is a very advanced field of chemistry and the synthetic abilities in this field both in terms of complexity of the synthesis as well as the scale-up of the processes are enormous.

Carbon can be obtained in nature in several forms. Until 1985, the known allotropic forms of carbon were amorphous, graphite, and diamond. This by itself sheds some light on the diversity of carbon organization at the molecular level, as graphite is one of the softest materials known in nature while diamond is of course one of the hardest. That implies that the precise molecular organization of the carbon can dramatically affect its macroscopic properties.

A new form of carbon was identified in 1985 by Curl, Smalley, and Kroto who shared the 1996 Nobel Prize in Chemistry for this discovery

Figure 2.3: The new form of C_{60} carbon clusters. The closed-caged buckminsterfullerene are formed by the arrangement of pentagons and hexagons into soccer-shaped closed cages.

(Kroto *et al.*, 1985). During experiments in which graphite was vaporized using a laser, new forms of carbon clusters were discovered. These clusters were in the form of fullerenes, closed and convex cage molecules formed by the arrangement of hexagonal and pentagonal faces (Figure 2.3). The most common and most stable carbon cluster was the buckminsterfullerene, named after the architect R. Buckminster Fuller due to the resemblance of the carbon structure with Fuller's geodesic domes. This caged cluster is a 60 carbon atoms spheroidal molecule, resembling a soccer ball in which hexagon carbons are arranged to form ordered closed structure pentagon carbon faces that serve as vertexes. Therefore, another popular name for the buckminsterfullerene is buckyball. This is in contrast to graphite, which is composed of a two-dimensional flat layer of hexagonal carbon arrangements. The C_{60} buckminsterfullerene is the most abundant cluster of carbon atoms found in carbon soot. Larger carbon fullerenes that have 70, 76, 84, 90, and 96 carbon atoms were also found to be formed under similar experimental conditions (Goel *et al.*, 2004).

The size of a C_{60} fullerene is about 0.7 nm and it shows excellent electrical and heat conductivity. Even smaller closed-cage carbon clusters are possible to obtain, including C_{50}, $C_{36,}$ and $C_{20.}$ The smallest possible fullerene, C_{20}, consisting solely of 12 pentagons, has been generated from a brominated hydrocarbon, dodecahedrane, by gas-phase debromination. Yet, the lifetime of the C_{20} was only about 0.4 milliseconds. It may be possible that in the future, ways will be found to stabilize these sub-nm structures. On the other hand, much larger carbon clusters are also found. Such closed-cage structures contain hundreds of carbon atoms. There were also descriptions of "carbon onions" in which, for example, a C_{20} was placed inside a C_{240} cage, which was in turn inside a C_{540} cluster cage.

Many applications have been suggested for the carbon fullerenes. Many of the biological or biotechnological ones are related to the ability of the assembly to serve as nano-containers for drug delivery or a reservoir to diagnostic agents. It was also demonstrated that modified fullerenes could serve as anti-viral agents. It was revealed that a modified C_{60} molecule could effectively inactivate HIV at low micromolar concentrations (Schinazi *et al.*, 1993).

2.5. Carbon Nanotubes: Key Building Blocks for Future Nanotechnological Applications

The discovery of the closed-cage carbon structures was followed by the discovery in 1991, by Sumio Iijima (Iijima, 1991), of a new form of carbon at the nano-scale, the carbon nanotubes. These nanotubes, in their single-shell form (known as single-walled nanotubes — SWNTs) are elongated variants of the C_{60} fullerenes that are described above. They practically resemble graphite sheets wrapped around into elongated cylinders with or without capping at their ends (Figure 2.4).

The formed nanotubes could be remarkably long. One key property of the carbon nanotubes is their remarkable aspect ratio: their length to width ratio is extremely high (few nm in diameter and up to 1 mm in length). Carbon nanotubes could also be formed in the multi-walled fashion (known as multi-walled nanotubes — MWNTs). In this arrangement the tubes are concentrically nested like rings of a tree trunk (Baughman *et al.*, 2002).

Carbon nanotubes have unique physical properties: both mechanical and electrical. They have a tensile strength that is about ten times greater than steel, yet at about one-quarter the weight. Therefore, carbon nanotubes are considered the strongest known material for their weight. As a result, carbon nanotubes are expected to be used in the development of ultra-strong materials for the construction, car, and aviation industries. Moreover, carbon nanotubes are envisioned as thread for ultra-strong

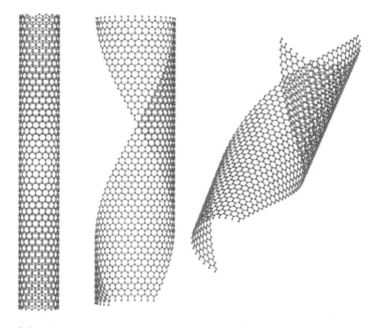

Figure 2.4: Model for the formation of carbon nanotubes by the two-dimensional graphite-like layer. The tubes presented here are single-walled, although double-walled and multi-walled carbon nanotubes also present. Courtesy of Dr. Chris Ewels (©Chris Ewels http://www.ewels.info/img/science/nanotubes/index.html).

fabrics and clothing such as lightweight bulletproof fabrics. One of the wildest ideas for the use of nanotubes is the assembly of an ultra-strong cable to be used for the construction of a space elevator.

Unlike a single sheet of graphite, which is a semiconductor, carbon nanotubes are found as a random mixture of conductive and semiconductive entities. The conductivity of the tubes depends on the direction by which the sheet of carbon is wrapped to form the tube. The conductivity of tubes on the one hand and their small size on the other led to the suggestion of the use of the tubes as molecular wires, conductive composites, and interconnects. Furthermore, the electric properties of carbon nanotubes appear to be modulated by various gases, for example nitrogen dioxide. Thus arrays of carbon nanotubes could serve as very sensitive gas sensors.

Other potential applications that have been proposed for carbon nanotubes include energy storage and energy conversion devices; field emission displays and radiation sources; hydrogen storage media; and nanometer-sized semiconductor devices (Baughman *et al.*, 2002; Collins *et al.*, 2001; Katz and Willner, 2004). As of 2011, many of these proposed applications have been demonstrated at the laboratory scale (Schnorr and Swager, 2011). It is worth mentioning that many of the potential commercial uses of carbon nanotubes are limited by their high cost of production. A pure sample of carbon nanotubes still costs, as of 2011, around 100 dollars a gram. Yet, many efforts are being invested in the construction of industrial settings for large-scale production of carbon nanotubes and their price is expected to be further lowered in the years to come.

2.6. A Single Layer of Carbon: Graphene

For a long time, it was believed that it was impossible to isolate a single sheet of carbon as a freestanding material. In 2004, Andre Geim, Konstantin Novoselov and colleagues succeeded in isolating thin flakes by repeated mechanical exfoliation of highly ordered-pyrolytic graphite (HOPG) platelets using a scotch tape (Novoselov *et al.*, 2004). They subsequently succeeded in transferring to a silica substrate and identifying flakes consisting only of one layer. A single layer of carbon, just one atom thick, was called graphene. Graphene has high thermal and electrical conductivity, and is a mechanically very strong yet stretchable material (Geim, 2009). Being transparent and conductive, it can be used in liquid crystal displays, solar cells, etc. Recently, uniform sheets of graphene of about 70 cm large could be produced (Bae *et al.*, 2010), and the ability to fabricate large sheets will enable industrial-scale applications in the future. Andre Geim and Konstantin Novoselov shared the Nobel Prize in Physics in 2010 for the discovery of graphene.

2.7. Non-Carbon Nanotubes and Fullerene-Like Material: The Inorganic Nanomaterials

As discussed in the previous section, carbon nanotubes are made of two-dimensional sheets of graphite that are rolled into a cylinder at the nano-scale. It is actually well known that not only graphite, but also inorganic materials such as WS_2, MoS_2, NbS_2 can form two-dimensional layered arrangements (Tenne, 2002). Therefore, in principle those

Figure 2.5: Transmission electron microscopy micrograph of MoS_2 fullerene-like nanoparticles. Courtesy of Dr. Reshef Tenne. Reproduced from Tenne, 2002, by permission of John Wiley and Sons.

structures could also be rolled to form either fullerene-like structures or nanotubes (Figure 2.6).

Indeed it was shown in 1992 by Reshef Tenne and coworkers that nanoparticles of the layered WS_2 compound can form closed-cage structures that are very similar in their molecular organization to carbon fullerenes and carbon nanotubes (Figure 2.6) (Margulis *et al.*, 1993). This instability was attributed to the highly reactive dangling bonds of both sulfur and tungsten atoms, which appear at the periphery of the nanoparticles.

This seminal work was followed by the demonstration of a variety of inorganic layered compounds such as MoS_2, $NiCl_2$, NbS_2, Tl_2O to form fullerene-like nanoparticles and nanotubes (Figure 2.6) (Tenne and Rao, 2004). It was therefore claimed that this nano-scale arrangement is generic to layered materials and numerous others. The production of inorganic nanomaterials has already become industrial and many technological applications were suggested for these materials. One of the most intriguing uses of these compounds is their application as solid lubricants. These fullerene-like inorganic nanomaterials have remarkable lubrication properties, which could significantly increase the lifespan and efficiency of

Figure 2.6: Transmission electron microscopy of WS_2 nanotubes. Courtesy of Dr. Reshef Tenne. Reproduced by permission from Macmillan Publishers Ltd. [*Nature Nanotechnology*], Tenne, R. (2006) Inorganic nanotubes and fullerene-like nanoparticles. *Nature Nanotechnol.*, **1**, 103–111. Copyright 2006.

motors and other power tools with moving parts. Indeed the application of these nanoparticles as additives for motor oil is currently being tested by major car manufacturers. Other applications, which are more relevant to biological applications, include their use as lubricants of medical and dental devices.

2.8. Quantum Dots and Other Nanoparticles

Other very intriguing assemblies at the low nanometric range are the quantum dots also known as nanocrystals (Empedocles and Bawendi, 1997). These nano-objects consist of semiconductor materials such as CdSe, CdTe, PbS, and PbSe surrounded by a shell that is usually composed of ZnS or CdS. These nano-assemblies have typical dimensions between a few nanometers to a few tens of nanometers (a few tens of atoms — a 10 nm core is composed of about 50 atoms), but could also be larger. The quantum dots basically serve as a cage for electrons, and the molecular diameters of these structures reflect the number of electrons they contain. A typical quantum dot can have anything from a single

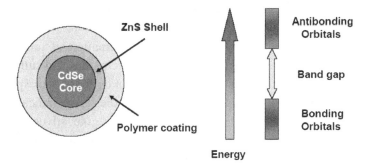

Figure 2.7: The organization of fluorescent quantum dots. The quantum dots are composed of a semiconductor core surrounded by a shell structure that is usually coated with polymers to give them specific properties (e.g., negative or positive charge or functional chemical groups). The fluorescence properties of the quantum dots arise from the energy gap of the confined electronic structures.

electron to a collection of several thousands depending on their specific size. The quantum dot basically behaves like a giant atom. As in a regular atom, the energy levels in a given quantum dot become quantized due to the confinement of electrons (Figure 2.7). The band gap between the two energetic states of the giant atoms determines the energy of a photon that is being emitted by the transition between states. The energy of the photons can be either in the visible or the infrared region depending on the specific band gap.

While quantum dots are extremely interesting from the physical point of view, for the purpose of this book the most important property is their fluorescent nature. A given quantum dot exhibits high fluorescent brightness that is stable and long lasting, while having narrow emission span. The exact emission wavelength of a given quantum dot depends on its physical diameter. Commercially available quantum dots have emission wavelengths ranging from the visible 465 nm to the 2300 nm infrared region. Their exceptional fluorescence properties distinguish them from conventional fluorescent dyes used in biology; however, the lack of aqueous solubility used to be a common barrier in their use for biological applications. This has been recently circumvented through the development of ligand exchange and coating techniques. Such soluble Q-dots functionalized with antibodies, proteins, or peptides are increasingly used in intracellular targeting and biological imaging applications (Jin *et al.*, 2011).

2.9. Nanowires, Nanorods, and Other Nanomaterials

In the previous section we discussed the formation of tubular and spherical nanostructures by carbon and inorganic oxides and sulfides. In all cases, layered materials wrap around to form cylindrical or spherical structures. In parallel to these works, other studies have indicated that many materials including metallic elements such as gold, silver or copper as well as single element semiconductors (such as silicon or germanium), compound semiconductors (such as InP, CdS and GaAs as well as hetero-structures), nitrides (such as GaN and Si_3N_4) to carbides (such as SiC) can form various ordered structures at the nano-scale. Such structures include small spherical nanoparticles, nanowires, nanobelts, nanoribbons, and nanorods. All these materials, especially the quasi-one-dimensional materials — wires, ribbons, and rods — have been attracting great research interest.

2.10. Magnetic Nanoparticles

The conductive and semiconductive nanomaterials attract much attention due to their potential use in nano-scale electronics. Yet, of many other applications, in high-density data storage there is a need for magnetic particles. Indeed, different magnetic nanocrystals were prepared from metal oxides such as MnO, CoO, Fe_2O_3, $MnFe_2O_4$ and $CoFe_2O_4$. The size of the nanocrystals can be as small as five nanometers. Furthermore, recent studies have demonstrated the ability to form a single 30 nm crystalline magnetite (Fe_3O_4) nanotube (Liu *et al.*, 2005). Some research is focused on the coating of metallic magnetic nanoparticles with various organic materials. One example is the use of lipid coating with results in water-soluble magnetic nanoparticles. Magnetic nanoparticles are very useful both as the media for storage as well as part of nano-scale reading heads. Another very important application of magnetic nanoparticles is their use as contrast agents in magnetic resonance imaging (MRI). This will be further discussed in Chapter 8.

Chapter 3

Natural Biological Assembly
at the Nanometric Scale

The process of self-assembly is central to all biological systems. All living cells evolve from simple building blocks which spontaneously self-associate into complex networks, molecular machines, and cellular structures. This is true for all organisms, from the very simple bacteria that have only a few hundred types of proteins for the building of their various nano-scale machines and assemblies, to mammals that have tens of thousands of different and varied protein building blocks as part of their molecular arsenal. Sophisticated molecular machines, such as the ribosome, composed of tens of protein and ribonucleic acid (RNA) molecules which assemble into highly ordered and well-defined structures, is a key example of a hierarchical self-assembly of a nano-machine from rather simple building blocks. In this chapter we will provide some background on the process of self-assembly and self-organization in biological systems. We will describe supramolecular biological assemblies that have both physiological as well as pathological roles.

3.1. The Process of Self-Assembly and Self-Organization in Biology

Self-organization of supramolecular assemblies is the central theme of biological systems (Whitesides *et al.*, 1991; Lehn, 2002). Unlike man-made engineered structures, complex three-dimensional biological systems are being spontaneously formed upon the association of simple building blocks into complex structures (Figure 3.1). The term "bottom-up", which was mentioned in the previous chapter as a future direction for nanotechnology, has been the natural choice for all living organisms. The "top-down" approach is the usual tool for conventional micro techniques.

Figure 3.1: The hierarchal process of self-assembly into complex structures. The formation of order assemblies at the nano-scale can work either by the "bottom-up" organization of molecules to form an ordered structure or by the engineering of a preformed pattern to serve as a template for molecular organization.

In most cases, the assembly of complex biological systems is not based on any prearranged templates, as we often see in engineering applications, but rather occurs through a process of molecular recognition and self-assembly events in which relatively simple building blocks recognize each other in solution, associate with one another, then associate with other molecules to finally form a well-organized three-dimensional functional entity (Figure 3.1).

3.2. Organization of Bacterial S-Layers

One fundamental feature of carbon and inorganic nanomaterials, as discussed in Chapter 2, is the organization of these materials into well-ordered crystalline or nearly crystalline forms of one-dimensional, two-dimensional, and three-dimensional order. Such organization of biological materials into ordered and crystalline nanomaterials can also be observed in several living systems. As will be demonstrated later in this book, these bio-assemblies are already used in technological applications.

A key example, which was already suggested for nanotechnological applications many years ago, is the two-dimensional bacterial S-layer assemblies. In a pioneering work, the structure, organization, and technological application of these assemblies were studied by Uwe B. Sleytr and co-workers (Schuster *et al.*, 2005). S-layers are bacterial cell surface structures that are found in all archaea and in hundreds of different species of walled bacteria (Figure 3.2). Archaea, as may be known to some readers, is a very unique group of prokaryotes which includes some extreme thermophilic and halophilic prokaryotes (DeLong and Pace, 2001). This interesting group of prokaryotes is phylogenetically distinct

Figure 3.2:   The S-layer structure. Transmission electron micrograph of a freeze-etched, metal-shadowed preparation of a bacterial cell with an S-layer with hexagonal lattice symmetry. The bar represents a distance of 100 nm. Courtesy of Dr. Uwe Sleytr. Reproduced from Pum, D., Neubauer, A., Gyorvary, E., Sara, M., and Sleytr, U. B. (2000) S-layer proteins as basic building blocks in a biomolecular construction kit. *Nanotechnol.*, **11**, 100–107, by permission from IOP Publishing Ltd. doi: 10.1088/0957-4484/11/2/310

from bacteria and has some similarity to eukaryotes, especially in their transcription and translation. Many of the organisms that belong to this group are extremophiles (organisms that require extreme conditions) such as halophiles ("salt-loving" organisms which could survive salt solutions of several molars such as in the Dead Sea) and thermophiles ("heat-loving" organisms that could survive temperatures higher than 100 °C). The adaptation of archaea and also some bacteria to such extreme environments may allow their application into stable nanotechnological devices for long-term usage, as the stability of common biomolecules is one of the limiting factors for their applications.

As the assembly of S-layers have been optimized through billions of years of evolution, it is one the most well-organized and highly efficient biological self-assembling systems. These two-dimensional layers are composed of single protein or glycoprotein species that assemble into an ordered layer which completely covers the cell surface. This layer exhibits clear lattice symmetry with spacing of the assembly units in the range of 3–30 nm. The thickness of the S-layers is at the nano-scale and ranges from 5–15 nm. They also possess pores of a seamless size and morphology in the 2–6 nm range. The very elegant use of these nano-scale ordered structures for nanotechnological applications will be described in Chapter 7.

3.3. Self-Organization of Viruses

Another well-studied biological process of self-assembly that was suggested for nanotechnological applications is the spontaneous template-assisted formation of viral shells. Viruses and bacteriophages (virus that infect bacteria — from "bacteria" and Greek *phagein*, meaning "to eat") are very abundant in nature and represent the simplest form of autonomous biological systems. Although viruses obviously need the cellular machinery of the infected hosts for their replication, they still represent an independent system which carries its own genetic information in a closed-caged environment. The defined molecular space which is isolated from the external world is a crucial element in self-replicating biological systems and represents the most fundamental aspect in the transition from a molecular collection into a living system. As will be discussed later in this chapter, it is usually achieved by the formation of lipid membranes for living organisms.

Figure 3.3: The formation of ordered tobacco mosaic virus (TMV) particles by the self-assembly of protein building blocks onto the RNA template. The RNA template serves as a pattern for the organization of the protein molecules to form a well-defined multi-component structure at the nano-scale.

The most intensively investigated viral assembly is that of the tobacco mosaic virus (TMV; Figure 3.3). TMV was the first macromolecular structure to be shown to self-assemble *in vitro* in 1957. In a classic work, Fraenkel-Conrat and Williams showed that upon incubation of the viral purified coat proteins and its RNA, virus particles formed spontaneously (Fraenkel-Conrat *et al.*, 1957). As will be described later for the ribosome, the specific interaction between the RNA nucleic acid and the proteins, results in the formation of well-ordered three-dimensional structures. This observation suggested that all the molecular information needed for the precise assembly of the virus is retained within the building blocks. Furthermore, as the structure is formed spontaneously without the supply of any external energy, such as high-energy nucleotides (for example, adenosine triphosphate (ATP)), as will be discussed for other forms of self-assembly later in this chapter, this clearly indicates that the self-assembled structure represents a minimal free-energy supramolecular structure.

The first studies on the structure of TMVs were performed in the 1950s using electron microscopy techniques which were beginning to be established and revolutionized biological research in many senses. These particles are seamless, rigid, rod-like structures that form a hollow cylinder of about 300 nm in length, an inner diameter of 4 nm, and an outer diameter of 18 nm. Each viral particle contains more than 2,000 protein subunits that are arranged as a right-handed helix. The RNA molecule is retained between successive turns of the protein helix. The process of TMV self-assembly starts with the binding of a bilayer disk of protein building blocks to a site on the viral RNA scaffold. Upon binding of the RNA, the protein subunits of the disk undergo a coordinated rearrangement to yield a helical nucleoprotein complex.

As with the S-layers, the TMV viral nanoparticle is a very interesting template of bionanotechnology. Its three-dimensional structure resembles many of those formed by inorganic or carbon nanostructures. Yet, unlike many of the pure carbon and inorganic nanostructures, these nanoparticles are formed spontaneously by self-assembly under mild conditions. Indeed, there were some reports on the metallization of TMV particles using electroless deposition (Knez *et al.*, 2003; 2004). Since then, reports continue to appear on genetically modified TMV protein units targeted for the templating of inorganic materials and applications at the nanoscale. We will further elaborate on these in Chapter 7.

Another form of well-ordered viral assembly is the formation of closed-caged structures composed of planar subunits that are closed together. This form of structure is known as icosahedral capsids, based on the symmetry of this platonic solid composed of identical subunits (Figure 3.4). Such capsids, e.g., the bacteriophage φX174, are built up

Figure 3.4: The formation of an icosahedral viral capsid by the self-assembly of protein building blocks into triangular elements that specifically interact to form the closed-caged assembly.

by using three identical protein subunits to form each triangular face, thereby requiring 60 subunits to form a complete capsid. The readers should note the similarity between the organization of the icosahedral capsid composed of triangular faces and the quasi-icosahedral C_{60} carbon fullerene composed of hexagons and pentagons. It should be noted that the combination of progress in crystallography and high-resolution electron microscopy techniques nowadays offers advanced structural knowledge on complex viral capsids. This is particularly illustrated by the appearance of atomic resolution structures of human adenovirus capsids in 2010 (Liu *et al.*, 2010; Reddy *et al.*, 2010). We will further elaborate on the use of viral capsids as nano-containers for inorganic material templating and biomedical applications in Chapters 7 and 8.

3.4. Self-Organization of Phospholipid Membranes

A self-assembly process which is crucial to any living organism is the spontaneous formation of lipid bilayers from phospholipid building blocks (Figure 3.5). Just like carbon and inorganic fullerenes, biological membranes are two-dimensional layers that are closed in space to form

Figure 3.5: The formation of liposome membranes by the self-assembly of phospholipids in aqueous solution. The driving force for the formation of the assemblies is the amphipathic nature of the phospholipid building blocks.

closed-cage spheroid structures. The main driving force of the formation of lipid membranes is hydrophobic interactions.

The phospholipid building block is an amphiphilic molecule which has a hydrophilic part, the phosphate head group, and a hydrophobic aliphatic tail. Upon transfer of phospholipid molecules into aqueous solution, a rapid and spontaneous association of the molecules occurs due to the enormous energetic cost of the presence of the aliphatic tail in water. The phospholipids organize into bilayer structures in which the aliphatic parts of each layer are pointed towards each other and the hydrophilic heads are pointed either to the bulk water or to the inside part of the closed structure.

The similarity of these structures to those presented in Chapter 2 is not limited to the closed-cage organization. Upon drying of the phospholipids from the hydrophobic organic solvent and their resolvation in water, "onion-like", larger multilamellar vesicles (LMV), of micron-scale dimensions are formed. Yet these "multi-walled" biological structures can be easily converted to small unilamellar vesicles (SUV) of single bilayers with sizes that range from a few hundreds of a nanometer to 50 nm upon sonication of extrusion. As with the rest of the layered materials, phospholipids can also form other organizations at the nano-scale; the more common one is the hexagonal phase of phospholipids. Yet, tubular structures, similar to the nanotubes mentioned in Chapter 2, can be formed by phospholipids under certain conditions (Figure 3.6). The ultrastructural analysis

Figure 3.6: Formation of lipid nanotubes by the self-assembly of glucopyranosylamide lipids. The driving forces for the formation of the structures are as presented in Figure 3.5, but the specific properties of the hydrophilic head group modulate the final morphology of the formed assemblies. Courtesy of Mitsutoshi Masuda. Reproduced with permission from Kamiya, S., Minamikawa, H., Jung, J. H., Yang, B., Masuda, M., and Shimizu, T. (2005) Molecular structure of glucopyranosylamide lipid and nanotube morphology. *Langmuir* **21**, 743–750. Copyright (2005) American Chemical Society (ACS).

of these lipid nanotubes by electron microscopy (Yager *et al.*, 1984; Yamada *et al.*, 1984; Nakashima *et al.*, 1985) reveals their similarity to the carbon and inorganic nanotubes described in Chapter 2. These are hollow structures with sub-micron diameters which are assembled due to the same physical principles that direct the formation of the bilayer structures. Thus, it is the free-energy-driven spontaneous formation of well-ordered structures that is based on the closure of two-dimensional layers into a closed structure.

The formation of either tubular or spherical structures is based on the geometrical properties of the building blocks, the relative dimensions of the hydrophilic and hydrophobic parts, as well as the conditions of molecular assembly. Readers should note that the common characteristics of the formation of alternating spherical and nanotubular structures between carbon and inorganic nano-structures (Chapter 2), as well as the lipid nano-structures presented here, will be recalled for the aromatic peptide structures in Chapter 6.

Small lipid vesicles, also known as liposomes, are well-studied nanoparticles. Even before nanotechnology became a fashionable field of research, many studies have been conducted on the use of liposomes as vehicles for drug delivery; one of the best examples of which is DOXIL®. This is a liposome injection of the anti-cancer drug, doxorubicin, which is successfully used to treat several forms of cancer with better efficacy and lower side effects, compared with the parent drug.

There is a great interest in the use of decorated SUVs as targeted drug delivery agents. The basic premise is to conjugate some type of targeting moieties, for example a cancer cell receptor, to a vesicle that contains chemotherapy agents. This should allow more effective treatment with a much lower degree of side effects. Interestingly, liposomes are already used in the cosmetic industry where it is claimed that they help to transport agents such as vitamin E and other antioxidants upon the penetration of the vesicles into the inner parts of the human skin.

3.5. Fibrillar Cytoskeleton Assemblies

Other ordered biological assemblies in the nano-scale are the building blocks of the cytoskeleton, a complex network of protein filaments which extends throughout the cytoplasm and serves as the physical and mechanical support of the cell, as well as intracellular cables for cargo movement. The cytoskeletal cellular main fibrillar elements are actin filaments, microtubules, and intermediate filaments which are all fibers at the nano-scale. These cytoskeletal elements facilitate the ability of cells to adopt a variety of three-dimensional shapes and to carry out coordinated and directed movements. The mechanical rigidity of the cytoskeleton elements was determined at the nano-scale using atomic force microscopy (AFM) techniques (de Pablo *et al.*, 2003). By physical measurement of the force needed to deform these structures their stiffness (represented as Young's modulus, named after the English physicist Thomas Young, the stiffness to withstand a physical load) was determined to be in the order of GPa, which is high compared with other nano-scale ordered structures.

Actin filaments (also known as *microfilaments*): These filaments are ubiquitous to all eukaryotic cells and the building blocks of the filaments, the actin proteins, are well conserved in evolution. Earlier analogues of actin, the FtsZ proteins, are found in bacteria, and also have structural roles in prokaryotic organisms. These are two-stranded helical polymers with a diameter of about 7 nm (Figure 3.7). They are quite flexible structures that are organized into a variety of linear bundles. The actin filaments are the

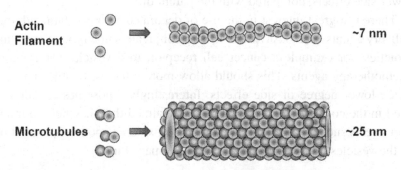

Figure 3.7: The major cytoskeleton nano-scale assemblies. The actin two-stranded helix is formed by the self-assembly of monomeric actin building blocks and has a diameter of about 7 nm. The microtubules are formed by the self-assembly of the tubulin dimeric building blocks into assemblies of about 25 nm in diameter.

principal components of the thin filaments in skeletal muscles and they have a key role in cell motility.

Microtubules: These are hollow cylinders with an external diameter of about 25 nm which are composed by polymerization of the tubulin protein building blocks (Figure 3.7). The microtubules are much more rigid when compared with the actin filaments. The microtubule network is attached to a central cellular entity known as the centrosome. Motor proteins, such as kinesin and dynein move along the microtubules to transport all kinds of cargo within the cell. While kinesin moves only in an "outbound" direction away from the centrosome, dynein is the "inbound" train moving only towards the center of the cell.

Intermediate Filaments: These filaments have ropelike cellular fibers with a diameter of about 10 nm. Their name comes from their intermediate dimension which is higher than the actin microfilaments and lower than that of the much larger microtubules. Unlike the actin filaments and the microtubules which are each composed of a single protein building block, actin and tubulin respectively, these intermediate filaments consist of a large and heterogeneous family of proteins. These filaments have diverse roles such as mechanical support for the cell and the formation of a network around the nuclear membrane.

Cytoskeleton polymers have already been used for nanotechnological applications. Actin filaments have been chemically reacted to covalently bind silver nanoparticles (Patolsky *et al.*, 2004a). The modified filaments were disassembled, excess silver was removed from the labeled monomers, and then the labeled monomers were reassembled either with labeled or non-labeled co-monomers. These labeled monomers, with the reassembled monomers, were used as nucleation sites for catalytic enlargement of the nanoparticles with gold. The enhancement process yielded gold wires (1–4 μm long and 80–200 nm high) that had very good electrical conductivity (Patolsky *et al.*, 2004a). Furthermore, the ATP-fueled motility of the actin-Au wire-actin filaments on a myosin interface was also demonstrated (Patolsky *et al.*, 2004a). This provided a vivid demonstration for the use of biological templates in the fabrication of inorganic materials at the nano-scale.

3.6. Nucleic Acids: The Genetic Information Media and a Template for Nanotechnological Applications

While most readers are familiar with the double helical structure of DNA (deoxyribonucleic acid) as was suggested by Watson and Crick in 1953 (for which they won the 1962 Nobel Prize in Physiology or Medicine), for quite a long time it was not considered as a typical nanomaterial. Yet, DNA is a typical well-ordered structure at the nano-scale. It has a diameter of about 2 nm and a length that ranges from a few nm to many microns (the distance between each base pair is 0.34 nm). DNA is a self-assembled structure that is spontaneously formed by two complementary stands in which cytosine (C) moieties interact with guanine (G) moieties and thymine (T) interact with adenine (A). All of these structures occur through a process of self-assembly. The overall structure is stabilized by aromatic base-stacking as appears in other bionanostructures as will be discussed later.

Ribonucleic acid can also form complex structures at the nano-scale. Yet, these structures are usually single-stranded structures in which intra-molecular, rather than intermolecular, interactions direct the formation of the complex three-dimensional structures of RNA, such as the transfer RNA (tRNA) molecule and structural building blocks of the ribosome nanomachine.

Much of the pioneering work on the use of DNA as a building material for nanostructures was performed by Nadrian Seeman, at New York University (Seeman, 2005). As will be described in more detail later in this book (Chapter 6), Seeman was able to demonstrate that complementary DNA strands could be designed to form complex two-dimensional and even three-dimensional cubic structures at the nano-scale. DNA appears to be a very attractive material for nanotechnology due to its relative thermal stability compared with protein building blocks. Moreover, the genetic engineering revolution very significantly advanced the field of DNA chemistry. It is now possible to synthesize very large DNA oligomers in high quantities, with a variety of chemical modifications and at relatively low cost.

Another very important work which established DNA as a nanotechnological material consisted of using it as a template for the fabrication of metallic nanowires (Braun *et al.*, 1998). This will also be further elaborated and illustrated in Chapter 6. Briefly, DNA molecules were coated with silver to form conductive nanowires. The same group went one step further to perform protein-based lithography on DNA templates (Keren *et al.*, 2002). In this case, a DNA-binding protein, RecA, was used to protect specific parts of the molecule from metal deposition and thus allowed a sequence-specific modification of the DNA template. In principle, through the design of exact recognition sites within a given DNA oligomer, a very specific pattern of metallization could be obtained.

Small oligonucleotides can assume a structural and even functional role. It was demonstrated that small RNA molecules, known as ribozymes, can have enzymatic activity as in the case of some RNA elements of the ribosome. Later studies have confirmed the ability of other small RNA and DNA molecules to carry out various enzymatic activities and the ability of small nucleic acid oligomers, known as aptamers, to serve as specific binders of various ligands.

3.7. Oligosaccharides and Polysaccharides: Another Class of Biological Polymers

The oligosaccharides and polysaccharides are polymeric chains in which sugar molecules are joined together by the formation of glycosidic bonds, upon the reaction of an aldehyde or ketone of one sugar molecule with the hydroxyl group belonging to another sugar. Small poly-sugar molecules are known as oligosaccharides in either branched or non-branched fashion. For example, glycogen is a long oligomer which is composed of glucose monomers joined together to form large and branched polymers. Most homogenic saccharides are used as a source for energy conservation. Yet, complex polysaccharides such as peptidoglycans, in which saccharides are complexed with a peptide template, serve as mechanical structures at a nano-scale order that maintains the mechanical properties of bacterial cells. Different oligosaccharides also have roles in the molecular recognition of the immune system and various bacteria, as specific antibodies are raised against specific polysaccharide structures. The exploration of oligosaccharides for specific nanotechnological uses is still to be made, but it may actually represent a very important direction in the future.

3.8. Amyloid Fibrils as Self-Assembled Nano-Scale Bio-Assemblies

The self-assembled structures as described in this chapter are mostly functional assemblies in living organisms. Another class of self-assembled structures was initially discovered as a pathological one. Yet, it plays a central medical role as well as an emerging role in the field of nanobiotechnology.

Amyloid assemblies are nano-scale fibrils which are characteristic of a large group of diseases of unrelated origin. A partial list of amyloid-associated diseases includes: Alzheimer's disease, type II diabetes, primary and secondary amyloidosis, and prion diseases (such as BSE — bovine spongiform encephalopathy, also known as "mad cow disease"). These assemblies can be found in various tissues and organs depending on the specific disease (e.g., in the brains of Alzheimer's disease patients or in the pancreas of type II diabetes patients).

Ultrastructural analysis of the amyloid assemblies using electron microscopy (EM) and AFM indicate that the deposits have typical 7–10 nm diameter fibrillar morphology, and a length of several micrometers. Furthermore, the observed fibrils are highly ordered with a clear meridional reflection in X-ray fiber diffraction patterns of about 4.6–4.8 Å and an equatorial reflection at about 10 Å. This pattern reflects a β-sheet secondary structure in which the β-stands perpendicular to the fibril axis, termed "cross-beta"; another tinctorial characteristic of these fibrils is a strong birefringence upon staining with Congo red dye. The regularity of the formed fibrils along their long axis, together with the classical nucleation and growth mechanism, has led to the reference of the process of amyloid formation as "one-dimensional crystallization" (Jarrett and Lansbury, 1993).

While amyloid-fibril nano-assemblies were previously considered to have only a pathological role, recent studies clearly demonstrate that the amyloid phenomenon may actually represent a significant physiological process. The first indication for such a role was the demonstration that biofilm formation by the *Escherichia coli* bacteria is facilitated by the self-assembly of the major curlin protein, CsgA, into typical amyloid fibrils (Chapman *et al.*, 2002). This finding was a milestone in the establishment of the notion that amyloid fibrils may act as functional physiological entities, and not only as pathological ones. It is also noteworthy that the characteristic diffraction pattern of the "cross-beta" structure was observed in 1968 for the fibrous stalks of the green lacewing fly, *Chrysopa flava* (Geddes *et al.*, 1968). The amino acid sequence of fibers from a fly endemic in Australia was only recently determined, revealing a silk-like fiber (Weisman *et al.*, 2009). A well-studied natural biomaterial exhibiting an amyloid structural signature are the chorion proteins, which form the eggshells surrounding silk moth oocytes (Iconomidou and Hamodrakas, 2008). These fibrous proteins confer mechanical strength and chemical protection. More recent studies revealed a role of amyloid structures in the formation of aerial hyphae by the *Streptomyces coelicolor* bacteria (Elliot *et al.*, 2003). In the last decade, reports keep appearing on natural materials with an amyloid-like structure, especially extracellular materials used for adhesion in algae, diatoms etc. (Larsen *et al.*, 2007; Mostaert *et al.*, 2006; Mostaert *et al.*, 2009). Amyloid self-assembly was also shown to play a role in the formation of yeast and fungi prions (King *et al.*, 1997). In these physiological phenomena, amyloids function as self-replicating structures which transmit genetic information and may confer evolutionary advantages in yeast physiology (True *et al.*, 2004; Greenwald and Riek, 2010). Functional roles for amyloids were also recently reported for mammals. In organelles called the melanosomes, amyloid fibrils are accumulated and serve as templates for the chemical synthesis of melanin, sequestering the highly toxic melanin precursors and preventing their uncontrolled release (Fowler *et al.*, 2006; 2007). Secretory granules seem to contain protein and peptide hormones in amyloid form, thus ensuring stable storage and release upon signaling (Maji *et al.*, 2008; 2009). Overall, these studies suggest that amyloid may be a structural pattern adopted by nature to play multiple roles in strength and protection, adhesion, or to serve as a storage and controlled release material (Knowles and Buehler, 2011; Otzen, 2010; Smith and Scheibel, 2010).

A major milestone in this important area of amyloid research was the emergence of atomic level structural information from several amyloid-forming peptides (Nelson and Eisenberg, 2006; Sawaya *et al.*, 2007). As we will extensively see in Chapters 6 and 7, amyloid-type structures are also emerging as structural and functional nanobiomaterials. Amyloid fibrils have already been demonstrated serving as building blocks for nano-electronics since part of a yeast prion protein which was genetically engineered was used as a template for the production of conductive nanowires. Engineered cysteine residues were used to bind gold nanoparticles along the self-assembled fibrils. An enhancement protocol was then used in order to obtain continuous conductive nanowires (Scheibel *et al.*, 2003) as will be further illustrated in Chapter 6. The recognition principles, as implicated in the formation of amyloid fibrils and most notably the key use of aromatic interactions, were later used in the design and fabrication of nanotubes and nano-spheres.

3.9. Silk: Natural Fibrillar Supramolecular Protein Assembly

The natural fibrillar supramolecular structures that are mostly related to amyloid fibrils, as discussed above, are those of spider and worm silk. These fibrils are predominantly composed of two protein molecules that create macroscopic filaments by precise molecular recognition and the self-assembly process (Kubic, 2002; Jin and Kaplan, 2003; Bini *et al.*, 2004; Eisoldt *et al.*, 2012). The notable properties of silk fibers are their outstanding strength and high flexibility. In spite of its non-covalent supramolecular nature, spider silk is considered to be on the one hand, remarkably stronger than a steel filament of the same diameter, but on the other hand highly flexible. These unusual mechanical properties are the basis for the stability and functionality of the spider's web and cocoon. This serves as a vivid example of the unique properties of supramolecular biomaterial, and its potential superiority over traditional organic and inorganic materials. The recombinant production of spider silk proteins in various organisms is a big challenge, due to their high molecular mass and repetitive nature of their sequences. However, recent work allowed their successful production in bacteria and their processing into fibers, spheres, and films which can be used mainly in tissue engineering and biomedical applications in general (Eisoldt *et al.*, 2011; Spiess *et al.*, 2010).

3.10. Ribosome: The Protein Assembly Line Instrument

The earlier examples in this chapter are mainly concerned with the formation of assemblies that either have a structural role or carry genetic information. Yet, the process of biological self-assembly can actually form functional machines. The most complex bionanomachine whose structure is known at the atomic resolution is the ribosome, the protein-RNA hybrid machine for the production of new proteins. The ribosome uses encoded data in the form of messenger RNA (mRNA) to form specific proteins, a process known as translation. The information for the identity of the protein is encoded in four letter — A, C, G, and T — triplet codes (known as codons). The 64 different combinations of the four letters represent a degenerate multiple code table, coding for the different 20 amino acids plus three codons that signal the translation process to stop. The coding molecule also includes information about the region of synthesis initiation.

The ribosome is a sophisticated self-assembled complex; it is a structure with a diameter of about 200 nm and consists of two subunits that fit together. Each subunit consists of one or two very large RNA molecules (known as ribosomal RNA or rRNA). A typical bacterial ribosome is composed of 55 different proteins and three RNA molecules. Structural insight on both subunits is available today at atomic resolution. Three structural biologists, Ada Yonath of the Weizmann Institute of Science, Venkatraman Ramakrishnan of the MRC Laboratory of Molecular Biology in Cambridge, and Thomas A. Steitz of Yale University, were awarded the 2009 Nobel Prize in Chemistry for their pioneering contributions to this remarkable achievement. The ribosomal functional assembly is formed by a spontaneous process of self-association. Indeed, if purified components of the ribosome are mixed together in a test tube, a functional ribosome can be formed. The route for self-assembly is a hierarchical and coordinated one. First, specific proteins bind the very large RNA molecules, which is followed by interactions of other proteins to finally form a ribosome of the original structure as well as function. This process resembles in some ways the self-assembly of the much simpler TMV as discussed previously in this chapter. As in the case of TMV assembly, the RNA molecules serve as templates for further coordinated, but spontaneously energy-favorable assembly of a much more complex structure.

3.11. Other Complex Machines in the Genetic Code Expression

As mentioned above, much is known about the main protein synthesis machine. Yet, the order of the processes of transfer and duplication of genetic information are also mediated by rather complex assemblies. Various molecular machines mediate the duplication of the biological information media, the DNA, as well as its transcription into the ribosome input, the mRNA. Cellular proteins, known as transcription factors, serve as on and off switches for the expression of this data according to the correct external conditions, or specific differentiation stage of the cell in the case of complex multicellular organisms. Other cellular machines are responsible for the maintenance of the correct DNA composition by error-correction mechanisms. These complexes are responsible, for example, for the correction of radiation-induced damage of the DNA. Indeed, individuals whose correction machines are dysfunctional suffer from a high incidence of cancer.

3.12. Protein Quality-Control Machinery: The Proteasome

It is important to note that the formation of protein structures is not a one-way process. The proteins which are synthesized by the ribosome in the process of genetic information expression are dynamic biochemical species. Proteins can be degraded by the cellular machinery into their amino acid building blocks. The half-life of a typical protein ranges from a few minutes to several days. The degradation of the proteins is a well-coordinated process which is mediated by complex cellular machinery as was discovered by Avram Hershko, Aaron Ciechanover, and Irwin Rose, leading to the Nobel Prize for Chemistry in 2004.

Proteins that are destined for degradation are marked by a molecular protein tag known as ubiquitin. The tagged proteins, depicted as ubiquitinated, are then degraded by a complex molecular assembly known as the proteasome. The proteasome is a nano-machine which has the shape of an elongated cylinder with a diameter of about 10 nm and a length of several tens of nanometers. The proteasome accepts ubiquitinated protein substrates and uses ATP energy to break them into basic building blocks.

3.13. Biological Nano-Motors: Kinesin and Dynein

Biological systems can form nano-motors that are orders of magnitude smaller than any man-made ones. Two biological motors which were previously mentioned in this chapter are kinesin and dynein, known as microtubule-associated proteins (MAPs). These two biological motors travel along the microtubules to transport organelles, vesicles, or other components of the cytoskeleton along the tubules (Marx *et al.*, 2005). These transported entities are known as "cargo". The molecular motors move on the tubules like trains over railway tracks. As described later, each of the motors moves in different directions along the microtubules. Kinesins move cargo away from the centrosome (anterograde transport), while dyneins transport cargo toward the centrosome (retrograde transport).

The energy needed for the movement of the motor proteins along the micro tubules track is supplied by ATP molecules. The kinesin motor is much smaller and less complex than the dynein motor, with a molecular weight of 380,000 and over 1,000,000 for kinesin and dynein, respectively. Therefore, the kinesin complex was studied extensively. The kinesin molecule is organized into three domains: two large globular head domains which bind ATP and facilitate the movement which are connected by a long coiled-coil helix to a tail domain, which binds the cargo. Experiments performed with purified kinesin and microtubules revealed the molecular mechanism of movement; it was found that the motor moves in discrete 8 nm steps. Mechanical measurement had revealed that the motor exerts a force of about 6 pico-Newtons (pN, 10^{-12} Newtons).

3.14. Other Nano-Motors: Flagella and Cilia

Another form of mechanical movement in biological systems is related to the movement of cilia or flagella. These types of swimming devices are common to bacteria, protozoa, and sperm cells. The cilia-mediated movement of eukaryotic organisms is based on the same molecular machinery as the microtubules motor with dynein as the major motor unit. Also, in this case chemical energy is converted to mechanical energy at the nanoscale to support the movement of various elements.

Another type of biological nano-motor is the F0-ATPase motor. This type of motor is found in bacteria as well as in mitochondria, the energy powerhouse of eukaryotic cells, which is of prokaryotic origin. This protein complex is used for the synthesis of ATP in the case of mitochondria. A proton motive force directs the forward movement of the motor resulting in the production of ATP. In the case of bacteria, the very same motor structure allows the production of mechanical movement for which the energy is supplied by ATP hydrolysis.

3.15. Ion Channels: Nano-Pores of High Specificity

Another group of nano-scale functional assemblies are the membrane-embedded ion channels, already mentioned earlier in this chapter. This class of protein assembly forms, by a process of self-assembly within the membrane, a nano-scale filter that allows the very specific transfer of a certain type of ion but not others. The most common ion channels are the sodium channels, potassium channels, and calcium channels. These channels have a key role in the electrophysiological process in which the function of the muscle is controlled by the central nervous system.

Much of our current knowledge about the structural basis of the remarkable selectivity of ion channels at the nano-scale comes from the pioneering work of Roderick MacKinnon. MacKinnon, who was the first to crystallize and determine the high-resolution structure of an ion channel (Morais-Cabral *et al.*, 1998) was awarded the 2003 Nobel Prize in Chemistry for his outstanding achievement. This was followed by the structural determination of several more ion-channel assemblies. The structural information together with biochemical and biophysical data on the function of the channels, should allow the design of these selective nano-scale filters in the future.

These molecular assemblies are ubiquitous in nature and can be found in all organisms. In higher organisms there are multiple forms of each type of channel that could be modulated by various signals, including physical (voltage gated) and chemical (ligand gated). Thus, these are assemblies which can indeed be considered as nano-scale devices, opening and closing very precisely at the nano-scale upon external control. Due to these properties of the channels, there are many nanotechnological attempts to use existing natural channels for detection and sensing at the nano-scale. Other attempts are directed towards the design of artificial nano-scale channels.

The formation of pores within the membrane is also being used by various organisms as a toxic strategy (Parker and Feil, 2005). Such pore-forming toxins permeate the membrane by the formation of nano-scale pores which are embedded within the lipid membranes. The aberrant flow of ions across the pore finally results in cellular dysfunction and, often, cell death. Such toxin-based nano-pores have already been used for nanotechnological applications (Meller *et al.*, 2000). For example, the 2 nm α-hemolysin pore was used in the transfer of nucleic acid polymers across membranes. The application of transmembrane potential serves as a driving force for the translocation of the charged DNA or RNA molecules. The monitoring of the changes in the current, as is reflected during the transfer of the oligonucleotides across the pore, is envisioned for rapid sequencing of DNA samples with many applications in genomics and diagnostics (Meller *et al.*, 2000; Mathe *et al.*, 2005). As of 2011, nano-pore sensors are foreseen to be competitive with other DNA sequence technologies and to contribute to the lowering of sequencing costs (Venkatesan and Bashir, 2011).

NB. *For the three-dimensional visualization of structures of proteins, RNA, DNA and other molecules discussed in this chapter, the reader is referred to Proteopedia, a three-dimensional, interactive encyclopedia created by scientists in 2009 (www.proteopedia.org). Even large macromolecular complexes such as the ribosome can be visualized, helping to build a detailed structural understanding of biological structures.*

Chapter 4

Nanometric Biological Assemblies: Molecular and Chemical Basis for Interaction

The specific interaction between building blocks, a principle already put forward in this book, is the key for the execution of the assembly processes. In this chapter, a brief introduction to the chemical and molecular basis of recognition and association processes is presented. We would like to give some formal background regarding the molecular and chemical basis for the introduction of these concepts to readers with no formal background in chemistry. We will discuss the thermodynamic basis for interactions and consider its entropic and enthalpic parameters. We will also provide some insights on the kinetics of macromolecular complex formation and its relevance to the biological function.

4.1. Emergence of Biological Activity through Self-Assembly

The process of self-organization has been discussed in previous chapters. In the context of biological nano-machines and functional assemblies, it is related to the way in which each key complex and elaborate functionality are produced by spontaneous association of discrete biomolecular elements into well-ordered assemblies. The association of biological assemblies is usually sequential and not parallel. Thus, high affinity and the equally important remarkable specificity between biomolecular motifs, is essential in the formation of these structures by the sequential processes of molecular recognition and self-assembly which leads to the formation of complex nano-scale machines.

The recognition motifs are usually protein molecules or nucleic acids (both DNA and RNA), although as discussed earlier in this book, biological affinity and specificity could be facilitated by other biomolecules such as sugars and their polymeric form of polysaccharides. We will first discuss the basic concepts of molecular recognition, affinity, and specificity from the chemical point of view. This will serve as the theoretical basis for the understanding and the experimental determination of the processes of recognition and assembly which lead to the formation of the ordered structures as described here. In the next chapter, we will put these chemical rules in the context of biological recognition and the formation of specific biological assemblies such as nucleic acid complexes and receptor-ligand interaction.

4.2. Molecular Recognition and Chemical Affinity

The process of molecular recognition is a key concept in the study of supramolecular chemistry as the chemical basis for non-covalent interactions between defined molecular moieties. This is of course not limited to biological systems but describes the interaction between chemical entities in general. The term "molecular recognition" describes the ability of two or more molecules to interact with each other at high affinity and specificity. As was described in Chapter 2, it is one of the cornerstones of supramolecular chemistry which is by itself one of the major aspects of nanotechnology.

The affinity between discrete molecular assemblies is often defined by the dissociation constant (K_d) of the formed complex. The value of K_d quantitatively describes the intensity of the binding between two or more molecules. This value, which is constant for a given molecular system, is a thermodynamic equilibrium value that could be described by the following formula for a simple two-component system in which two molecules A and B form a dimeric complex (obviously in the case of a multiple component system, the mathematical expressions become more complex):

$$Kd = [A] \times [B] / [AB], \qquad (4.1)$$

where [A] and [B] are the molar concentrations in equilibrium of molecules A and B, respectively, and [AB] is the molar concentration of a bimolecular complex composed of A and B. As could easily be observed from the equation, the units of K_d for this simple bimolecular system are molars (abbreviated as M). The K_d is often attributed to the "affinity" of the macromolecular system; thus an "nM affinity" means a nanomolar $(10^{-9} M) K_d$ value.

It is worth noting that for many practical applications, it is often complicated to determine the exact concentration of all free molecular species. However, if the concentration of one of the molecules, let us assume B, is much lower than the concentration of A (i.e., [B]<<[A]), one can assume that at a given concentration the amount of added A ($[A_{total}]$) is almost equal to the amount of free A (denoted as [A]). Under these conditions the concentration of total A in which half of B is bound equals the K_d, as under these conditions:

$$[B] = [AB] \rightarrow K_d = [A] \sim [A_{total}].$$

This practical approach is often used to experimentally determine the values of K_d in a relatively simple way. Allowing a large difference between the concentration of A and B, molecule B is labeled with a very sensitive probe such as radioactive or high quantum-yield fluorescence labeling. Such experiments were used to determine the affinity between antibodies and antigens, DNA and DNA-binding protein, and receptors and ligands, as will be described in the next chapter.

Specific binding is usually attributed to K_d values which are lower than 10^{-6} M (1 μM), although as will be described below for specificity, the relative affinities are more important than the nominal value. High specificity binding between an antibody and antigens or a transcription factor and DNA are often in the nanomolar (10^{-9} M) range. However, the affinity could be even higher, as some antibody–antigen complexes have K_d values as low as 10^{-11} M. The strongest non-covalent biomolecular complex is that between avidin and biotin which is frequently used as a connecting adaptor in biotechnological and nanotechnological applications (Wilchek and Bayer, 1990). Since this avidin–biotin binding is so strong, it could not be determined accurately, but it is assumed to be in the order of 10^{-15} M which practically behaves as a covalent binding between atoms.

4.3. Affinity and Specificity of Biological Interactions

A strong affinity between two biomolecular entities is of course important but yet insufficient for high specificity. The specificity of biological interaction is defined by the relative affinity of a given molecule to its molecular target compared with non-specific targets. For example, in the case of DNA-binding proteins, that are often positively charged molecules, there is some non-specific interaction even with non-specific DNA fragments that are negatively charged polyanions. Yet, while the non-specific DNA-protein interactions are in the order of 10^{-3} to 10^{-4} M, the specific binding of the proteins to the correct molecular target is often in the range of 10^{-7} to 10^{-9} M. There are also other cases in which the same molecular receptor can bind different ligands in various affinities and thus modulate the biological activity of the complex by some combinatorial binding pattern.

A clear specificity is not limited only to the binding of simple complexes but can also be related to the specificity of ion channels, e.g., the transmembrane nano-channels described in Chapter 3, which allow the transport of specific ions but not others. One example is the potassium channel which allows the effective transport of potassium ions but not the very similar sodium ions. The specificity is reflected by the orders of magnitude difference in the transport rate between the two cations. Another biological specificity stems from the activity of enzymes that can distinguish between very similar substrates and catalyze unique chemical reactions. An example of this specificity is the activity of sugar-modifying enzymes that are critical for energy conversion cascades such as cellular glycolysis, which specifically and clearly distinguish between similar sugars such as glucose and fructose.

4.4. The Relation Between Thermodynamics and Kinetics
of Dissociation

While K_d is a thermodynamic parameter, it is of course directly linked to the kinetic properties of the complexation reaction (for a simple bimolecular dimeric system):

$$K_d = k_2/k_1, \qquad (4.2)$$

where:

k_1 (rate of dissociation) **AB ---> A+B**, and
k_2 (rate of association) **A+B --->AB**.

Thus, as k_2, the rate of association, is related to the concentration of the components of the complex, k_1 is independent of the concentration of the complex. While the rate of association is usually similar for various biomolecular partners of similar size and is directed by the rate of diffusion, the rate of dissociation is directly linked to the affinity of the complex. Due to this property, in many cases where there is a problem in having one of the molecular partners at a much lower concentration compared with the other one (as described in Equation 4.2), the rate of dissociation serves as a criterion for the molecular affinity. Many high-affinity complexes may have dissociation rates of hours or days, while low-affinity complexes may have dissociation rates of milliseconds or shorter.

If specific antibodies are available, the kinetic rates could be determined using common biological assays such as ELISA (enzyme-linked immunosorbent assay) in which the ligands are attached to multi-well plastic plates and the interaction is probed by antibodies. In other cases, the degree of complexation could be determined by colorimetric methods or fluorescence spectroscopy. However, in recent years there has been an increased tendency to use the surface plasmon resonance (SPR) technique for the determination of the binding kinetics between non-labeled species. There are several commercially available instruments that utilize the SPR technique, the most famous one is the Biacore®, but other commercial systems from other manufactures are available.

The basic principle of this technique is based on the immobilization of one of the interacting molecules onto the surface and measurement of the changes in the surface optical properties upon the binding of the second molecule. The surface plasmon is an electromagnetic surface-bound wave that propagates along the interface between a metal and a coating layer. In commercial instruments, a metal surface is modified with biological molecules and the changes in the reflective index upon binding are determined (Figure 4.1).

Figure 4.1: The use of SPR to monitor the kinetics of association and dissociation between biomolecules. The interaction between the molecules on the metal surface affects its optical properties. When the signal is plotted as a function of time, the kinetics of association and dissociation can be resolved.

During a typical SPR experiment, a solution containing the binding molecules is injected to the chamber which contains the other partner of the molecular pair that is bound to the surface. The real-time change in the resonance signal as a function of time is plotted. This plot, referred to as a "sensogram", gives information about the rate of association of the molecules. When the injection of the molecules is halted and only the vehicle solution is being injected, a dissociation process occurs, which could also be followed. As discussed above, when both the association rate constant as well as the dissociation rate constants are known, the thermodynamic K_d can be directly calculated. While SPR is a very useful method, it should be noted that it is useful when the immobilization of the molecules to the surface does not affect the binding reaction and when the injected molecules do not interact with the surface by non-specific adhesion or other interactions.

4.5. The Chemical Basis for Molecular Recognition and Specific Binding

The formation of complex non-covalent biological structures often stems from the combination of many small energy interactions in which the linear combination of their contributions together forms a complex structure of high affinity. Such interactions can include hydrogen bonds (relative energy of less than 1.0 Kcal/mol), van der Waals interactions, hydrophobic interactions, and electrostatic interactions. The overall free energy of interaction can be derived from the dissociation constant as:

$$\Delta G = RT \ln(K_d), \qquad (4.3)$$

where ΔG is the free energy of interaction, R is the gas constant, and T is the absolute temperature.

4.6. The Formation of Specific Complexes by an Increase in Entropy

As described in the previous section, the formation of high-affinity complexes is based on the free energy of association.

$$\Delta G = \Delta H - T\Delta S, \qquad (4.4)$$

where ΔH is the change in the enthalpy of interactions, and ΔS is the change in the entropy of interactions. A full description of thermodynamics is beyond the scope of this book. However, in quite a simplistic way

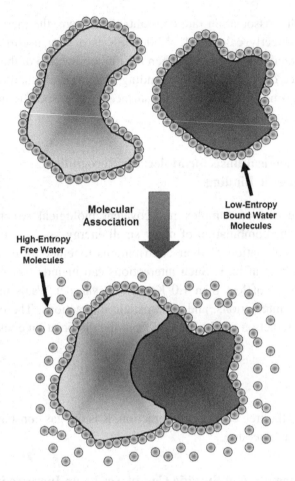

Figure 4.2: The molecular basis for association between macromolecules which is driven by entropy.

enthalpy could be described as the heat-related interaction, while entropy describes the disorder of the system. The actual contribution of entropy and enthalpy in the formation of biomolecular complexes could be determined by a special calorimetric technique known as isothermal titration calorimetry (ITC). This is a very sensitive calorimetric technique in which the heat generated upon specific molecular interactions is recorded upon the sequential addition, by injection, of a solution containing one molecule to a calorimetric cell that contains the other studied molecule.

The technique allows the determination of the enthalpy, ΔH, of the interaction and the K_d of binding. The experimental determination of the two parameters allows the calculation of the entropic part of the interaction reaction, ΔS, as described above.

The formation of a biomolecular complex appears intuitively as an event that results in an increase of order and thus a decrease in entropy. Yet, when many cases of complex formation are studied by calorimetry, they are actually driven by entropy rather than enthalpy. Thus, the formation of ordered complexes actually results in an increase in the disorder of the system. The explanation for this paradox is the fact that dissolved biological molecules in aqueous solution are actually surrounded by several layers of ordered water molecules (Figure 4.2). Upon the interaction of the biomolecules, ordered water molecules from the recognition interface are released to the bulk water which results in an overall increase in the disorder of the system.

Chapter 5

Molecular Recognition and the Assembly of Biological Structures

In the previous chapter, we provided some theoretical background regarding the kinetic and thermodynamic basis for the specific recognition between macromolecules. We have discussed some formal aspects of the association and dissociation both as a dynamic kinetic process as well as an equilibrium thermodynamic state. In the current chapter we will describe a few of the specific recognition and assembly processes that lead to the formation of ordered biological complexes. We will describe both the formation mechanisms of the biological complexes as well as some possible directions for their use in nanotechnological applications.

5.1. Antibodies as the Molecular Sensors of Recognition

The ultimate cellular entities which allow specific recognition of various compounds, organic and inorganic, biological and non-biological, are the antibody proteins. The unique recognition properties of these relatively large protein molecules allow a very high affinity of molecular recognition of various ligands. The K_d of the interactions of antibodies with a given ligand can reach the order of 10^{-12} M (picomolar) or even femtomolar (10^{-15} M) concentrations. Antibodies not only possess high affinity, but also high specificity as they can distinguish between extremely similar ligands. Antibodies are of course a key component of the immune system and have a crucial role in the protection of individuals against pathological states ranging from infections to malignant transformation. The description of the immune system mechanism is beyond the scope of this book, but those readers with no background in immunology are highly encouraged to further read about this remarkable system.

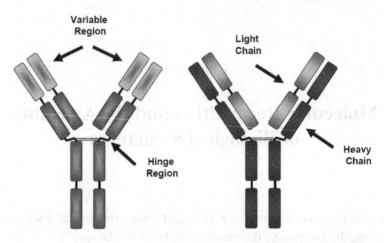

Figure 5.1: The basic structure of antibodies. The Y-shape structure is formed by the interaction of a heavy chain and a light chain. The specific recognition of the antibody molecules is facilitated by the unique structural features of the variable region.

Just as a brief overview, we would like to mention that the high affinity of antibodies is achieved by the selection of specific recognition interfaces for a set of complex combinatorial amino acid arrangements (Figure 5.1). Typically the Y-shape structure of an IgG (immunoglobulin G) antibody is made up of V (for variable) and C (for constant) regions. A hinge region in the middle of the IgG antibody confers flexibility on the molecule. The high binding of antibodies to their ligand is further increased by the avidity of the antibodies. The cellular antibodies contain more than one binding site for a given ligand. In the case of the IgG antibodies, the affinity is increased by the existence of two binding sites. There could be up to five identical recognition sites for the IgM antibodies; in this way, much stronger binding is achieved. The effect of the multiple binding sites could be intuitively understood by the consideration of the dissociation rate constants described above. In order for the antibody to be released from its molecular target, there is a need for release from the two binding sites at the same time. As the two or more dissociation steps are statistically independent events, the probability for antibody release is the product of the independent probabilities.

For the purpose of this book, we will describe the various technological applications of antibodies. The biotechnological uses of antibodies were mentioned in Chapter 1, as some of the common diagnostic kits, such as home pregnancy-test kits, are based on the use of the high specificity of antibodies and their ability to detect minute amounts of ligands in a complex mixture. The combination of antibodies together with nanotechnology tools could lead to even higher levels of sensitivity. One classic example is the development of the latest generations of home pregnancy kits which combine gold nanoparticles with an immunochromatographic test-strip assay. The test strip is coated with gold nanoparticles conjugated with a primary antibody against the pregnancy hormone mentioned in Chapter 1. In the presence of the hormone in the urine, the complex formed migrates by capillarity to a lane containing an immobilized capture antibody. The immobilization and concentration of gold nanoparticles appears as a red line. It was demonstrated that the conjugation of specific antibodies with DNA barcode magnetic nanoparticles could lead to attomolar (10^{-18} M) scale detection of the prostate-specific antigen (PSA) protein, a key indicator of prostate cancer (Nam *et al.*, 2003). This is a clear example of the great prospects of the combination of biotechnology together with nanotechnology for the ultra-sensitive bio-sensing. In the case of PSA this could lead to early detection of prostate cancer, yet the attainment of ultra-sensitivity could have ample application outside the medical field. One example is in environment monitoring and homeland security applications in which minute amounts of biological and chemical agents could be detected.

5.2. Selection of Antibodies and Equivalent Systems in the Test Tube

As mentioned above, antibodies are one of the most elaborate biological molecular recognition modules. The excellent affinity and specificity properties of antibodies encouraged the attempts to develop such systems in the test tube. Artificial libraries that contain antibody repertoires are being expressed by bacteria and after cycles of selection, high-affinity antibodies are produced. This allows the production of antibodies which have affinity and specificity even to "self" ligands or other entities with low antigenic potential. The field of antibody selection has advanced significantly in recent years. One of the most important directions is the engineering of single-chain antibodies. These antibodies should have many uses in further therapeutic applications.

Figure 5.2: Selection of specific binders by phage display techniques. Iterative cycles of enrichment are used to obtain high-affinity binders. The selection starts with a random library which is significantly enriched after only binder phages are retained and further used to infect bacteria.

Another means of achieving high-affinity biological systems is the use of phage display systems (Figure 5.2). In those systems, antibodies or other peptidic entities are presented on the surface of filamentous bacteriophages. Several cycles of binding and selection, known as panning, allow us to obtain phage particles that bind the molecular target at high affinity and specificity. Another direction for obtaining molecular recognition entities from non-living systems is the use of chemical peptide libraries. These libraries could have the molecular diversity of 10^{-12} or even higher, which can allow us to obtain small molecules that bind their target at relatively high affinity. While the disadvantage of the peptide libraries is the inability of sequential enrichment using cycles of panning, one of the advantages is the ability to use non-natural building blocks in the libraries. This of course allows us to significantly increase the chemical diversity and to obtain non-cleavable peptide entities. This is especially important for the therapeutic industry. The use of synthetic chemical libraries is of course not limited to peptides. Other organic, or even inorganic molecules, could be probed for their ability to bind various biomolecules.

The use of bacteriophages as building blocks for nanotechnology was demonstrated by the pioneering work of Angela M. Belcher and her co-workers. This will be described in detail in Chapter 7. Briefly, the nano-scale size of the bacteriophage building blocks together with the ability to engineer them with specific recognition abilities allows the formation of nanostructures with unique recognition properties.

5.3. Recognition between Nucleic Acids by Proteins

The recognition of specific DNA sequences by protein molecules known as DNA-binding proteins was mentioned earlier in this book. This specific recognition lays the basis of the complex control of the expression of the genetic information in various organs and tissues in multicellular organisms and under different growth conditions by microorganisms.

The DNA-binding proteins have the unique ability to recognize a specific sequence motif that could be as short as six or eight base pairs out of the millions or billions of base pairs in a given genome. In order to execute a correct molecular response, these proteins not only have to bind with high-affinity regulatory DNA motifs, but the specificity of interaction also needs to be high. The complex cascade of protein-DNA interaction that controls a biological complex was first demonstrated in the lactose operon of *E. coli*, but was later described in much more complex organisms including human cells.

One of the fascinating properties of DNA-binding proteins is their ability to recognize their specific binding sites very quickly and accurately out of millions of possible combinations. Although several high-resolution structures of protein-DNA complexes are already known, the exact way in which the protein finds its specific target is not fully understood. It is assumed that some non-specific binding of the protein to the DNA occurs by non-specific electrostatic interactions by either scanning the DNA strand or randomly moving from one site to another until a high-affinity binding site, which is reflected by very slow dissociation, occurs. Interestingly, careful biophysical analysis has indicated that the specific protein-DNA interaction may be facilitated by entropy rather than enthalpy (Garner and Rau, 1995). Thus, the non-specific initial binding is mediated by electrostatic interactions between the positively charged DNA-binding proteins and the polyanion DNA, while the specificity is modulated by the release of hundreds of water molecules upon the specific binding to the exact recognition site. The molecular basis for such mechanisms of specificity is explained in Chapter 4.

DNA-binding proteins such as the RecA protein have already been used for nanotechnological applications as will be described in Chapter 7. Briefly, the ability of the protein to bind a very specific site in the DNA with sub-nm precision is used for bio-lithography where the protein serves as a nano-scale mask on the DNA.

5.4. Interaction between Receptors and Ligands

Molecular recognition also serves the execution of biological function in the extracellular milieu. Various receptors are embedded in the cellular membrane and allow the response of the cells to various signals. The best studied receptors are those that recognize hormone signals. Hormones are used to carry biological signals through the blood stream and the recognition by the membrane receptor allows the correct biological response.

A paradigm for hormone receptors is that of the insulin receptor. The level of blood insulin is probed by membrane-embedded receptors in the periphery tissues. The recognition is mediated by a set of non-covalent interactions as described above for other supramolecular assemblies. The high affinity between insulin and its receptor allows sensitive sensing but a limited occupancy of the receptor site. The binding of the insulin to the insulin receptor results in the executing of a molecular cascade that ends up in the activation of specific genes which regulate the metabolism of sugars in the target cells.

The interaction between the receptors and ligands may also have nano-technological applications as the high affinity and specificity can allow the accurate assembly of subunits into nano-scale order assemblies, the modulation of activities of nano-devices and assemblies, and the use of these interactions for diagnostic purposes.

5.5. Molecular Recognition between Nucleic Acids

One of the most important specific recognitions between biological molecules is the interaction of complementary DNA and RNA strands. As most readers know, DNA is formed from four types of bases A, C, T, and G, and the molecular basis for the high specificity of DNA double-stranded structures derives from the specific affinity between A and T pairs and those made of C and G. The energy of interaction between single base pairs is quite small (three hydrogen bonds stabilize the CG pair and two hydrogen bonds stabilize the AT pair). Yet, in a typical double-stranded DNA when tens, hundreds, or thousands of base pairs are joined together, the overall chemical affinity is quite high.

DNA can also form specific heteromolecular complexes with RNA molecules. These interactions are based on the same recognition rules as described above. Yet, in the case of RNA molecules, the T base is substituted by the U base to form specific AU basepairs. RNA, and in some cases DNA, can form intermolecular base pair interactions to form complex three-dimensional structures at the nano-scale. The best known example is the formation of transfer RNA (tRNA) molecules.

The specific interaction between nucleic acid molecules is already used in several bionanotechnological applications. The specificity of nucleic acid interaction can serve as a very specific addressing entity or molecular barcode. Moreover, DNA molecules by themselves can serve as a template in the formation of two-dimensional and three-dimensional assemblies as was demonstrated by the pioneering work of Nadrian Seeman which will be described in Chapter 6.

5.6. Aptamers

Aptamers are short, single-stranded oligonucleic acids, composed of either DNA or RNA, which are able to adopt three-dimensional structures and can recognize with high specificity a variety of targets. These targets can range from small chemical molecules, biological simple building blocks (peptides, nucleic acids, saccharides) to biological macromolecules and even more complex targets such as viral particles and cells. They are identified by using *in vitro* selection processes, such as those described in Section 5.2. Using a process called SELEX (systematic evolution of ligands by exponential enrichment), the best binding candidates to the target molecule are selected from a library of 10^{15} nucleotide sequences after iterative cycles or enrichment and amplification. Aptamers therefore present the following advantages compared with antibodies: no use of animals is required, and aptamers can be generated even against toxic or non-immunogenic substances. Once the proper sequences are identified, they can be easily synthesized and even modified chemically, and lot-to-lot variability is not an issue. Therefore, aptamers present an increasing potential of applications in biosensing, diagnosis, and therapeutic applications (Lee *et al.*, 2010). To cite an example, an aptamer directed against VEGF (vascular endothelial growth factor) (Ng *et al.*, 2006) has obtained FDA approval and is currently used for the treatment of ophthalmological macular degeneration (www.macugen.com).

Chapter 6

Self-Assembly of Biological and Bio-Inspired Nanomaterials

In previous chapters we have described the formation of nano-structures in various biological systems, the thermodynamic and kinetic basis for the molecular recognition and self-assembly process, and some key examples for such recognition and assembly processes in physiologically relevant systems. In the current chapter we will describe the design of novel biological and bio-inspired building blocks which are based on the principles described earlier. These designed nano-structures have a great potential for both bionanotechnological and nanobiotechnological applications.

6.1. Formation of DNA-Based Materials

One of the earliest studied assemblies of ordered materials at the nanoscale was that of two-dimensional and three-dimensional DNA structures. The physiological basis for the interaction of DNA at the nano-scale was described in Chapter 2. Here we will describe the use of these principles. The pioneering work in this field was made by Nadrian Seeman a few decades ago before nanotechnology became such a central field (Seeman, 1990; 2005). Seeman, a crystallographer by training, had recognized the great potential of the molecular recognition and complementary of DNA oligomers, as were described in Chapter 3, to fabricate complex materials that are based entirely on molecular recognition and self-assembly processes (Figure 6.1). Long before nanotechnology became a major scientific discipline, Seeman had already manipulated DNA assemblies at the nano-scale to form complex and elaborated structures (Seeman, 1990).

Seeman had used DNA oligomers that have internal complementary recognition interfaces (Figure 6.1). When those DNA molecules were

Figure 6.1:　Self-assembly of linear DNA polymers into two-dimensional junctions. The interaction is based on the complementary nature of the single-stranded DNA molecules (1 and 1′, 2 and 2′).

mixed in aqueous solution, a spontaneous self-assembly process occurred which resulted in the formation of ordered two-dimensional arrays of DNA. Follow-up studies made the design into even more complex two- and three-dimensional structures, such as DNA cubes. A study from the same group had also used the DNA architecture to design DNA-based nanotubes (Sherman and Seeman, 2006; Wang *et al.*, 2012).

Since the early days of DNA-based materials many applications by various groups were developed (for a review see Feldkamp and Niemeyer, 2006). DNA oligomers have many advantages as molecular materials due to their high thermal stability compared with proteins (but not to peptides as will be discussed later in this chapter). Furthermore, the molecular biology revolution had created a great need for synthetic DNA oligomers for various reactions. This resulted in the optimization of the large-scale solid-phase chemical synthesis of DNA oligonucleotides (known in short as "oligos") and a significant decrease in the price of custom-made DNA. The price of DNA oligomers was reduced in orders of magnitude over a period of 20 years. Moreover, the need for various modified versions of DNA increased the chemical diversity of the commercially available DNA oligos. One of the disadvantages of the DNA assemblies is their sensitivity to enzymatic degradation by various nucleases which are ubiquitously present on most surfaces.

DNA is not only used by itself for the molecular assembly of nano-structures, but also as a template for the organization of other molecules such as proteins and peptides. Christof M. Niemeyer and co-workers had developed very intriguing applications of the specific recognition of DNA for the organization of proteins and inorganic nanoparticles to form various functional nano-devices (Feldkamp and Niemeyer, 2006). One of the interesting applications involves biotinylated DNA oligonu-cleotides which specifically bind avidin-modified surfaces. The remark-ably high affinity between avidin and biotin results in an extremely efficient organization of the molecular building blocks into highly ordered assemblies at the nano-scale. Such nano-patterned surfaces were also further modified by a metal coating in order to achieve func-tional electronic devices. As of 2012, the art of "DNA origami" (Rothemund, 2006; Sacca and Niemeyer, 2012; Seeman, 2010) can produce very elegant and complex three-dimensional shapes with prom-ising potential applications in energy transfer, diagnostics, therapeutics, etc. (Pinheiro *et al.*, 2011).

6.2. Assembly of Peptide-Based Nanomaterials

As with DNA molecules or oligomers, peptides represent another major group of biological macromolecules. Peptides, which are polymers of amino acids, are some of the most important and diverse biomolecules; synthetic peptides, which can be as short as a dipeptide but also as long as 40-mer polymers, are the most important and chemically diverse entities for nanotechnology applications (Zhang, 2003; Reches and Gazit, 2006a). Like DNA oligomers, peptides are also synthesized readily and efficiently by solid-phase methods. In fact, the chemical synthesis of peptides was demonstrated well before the synthesis of DNA oligomers. In the 1960s,

Bruce Merrifield and co-workers developed the solid-phase synthesis of peptides which has been practiced using similar principles up to the present day (Merrifield, 1965). For this seminal work, Merrifield was awarded the 1984 Nobel Prize for Chemistry.

One of the great advantages of peptides is their chemical diversity compared with nucleic acid oligomers. DNA oligomers are basically composed of only four different letters. Therefore, the chemical complexity of a given DNA oligonucleotide is 4^N, where N is the length of the oligonucleotide. On the other hand, the complexity of peptides which are composed of only the 20 natural amino acids is 20^N. Therefore, a large diversity is achieved even with very short peptides. For example, the chemical complexity of natural pentapeptides is $20^5 = 3,200,000$. The complexity of a 5-mer DNA oligomer is only $4^5 = 1,024$; more than three orders of magnitude lower. The actual situation is even more extreme as there are hundreds of non-natural amino acid monomers which are commercially available. Moreover, many termini modifications also exist; these modifications can significantly affect the biochemical and biophysical properties of the peptides. Therefore, the practical chemical space of a simple pentapeptide which also contains non-natural amino acids is more than 10^{10}.

Peptides can also be synthesized at the kilogram scale in a quite simple way and inexpensively for short peptides. The best example of a dipeptide which is synthesized on a very large scale is the aspartyl-phenylalanine methyl ester, also known as Aspartame™. This widely used sweetener is synthesized at a cost of a few cents per gram.

Short synthetic peptides corresponding to the building blocks used in natural proteins can very often self-assemble into either native-like or non-native hierarchical assemblies. The α-helix and the β-sheet are two basic "modules" of structure used to build protein architectures. In the α-helix, the polypeptide chain folds into a spiral-like conformation held, with hydrogen bonds, between the CO group of the amino acid i and the NH group of the amino acid i+4. In the β-sheet, the chain folds into an extended strand conformation and strands are connected with hydrogen bonds between amino acids which could be distant in the primary sequence. Understanding the structural rules which govern the assembly of natural building blocks further allowed the design of *de novo* building blocks that did not correspond to any natural protein sequence. As we will see below, their ability to self-assemble opened the way for the rational design of simple building blocks competent for supramolecular self-assembly.

6.3. The First Peptide Nanotubes

Peptides were recognized as excellent building blocks for nanotechnology in the 1990s. Peptides have the great advantages of chemical diversity and flexibility as described above, but also other advantageous properties for nanotechnology, including biocompatibility and stability.

One of the key pioneering studies on the use of peptides as structural elements at the nano-scale was the synthesis of the first peptide nanotubes by M. Reza Ghadiri and co-workers (Ghadiri *et al.*, 1993). The researchers demonstrated the formation of hollow nanotubular assemblies by the self-assembly of cyclic peptides, designed with an even number of alternating D- and L-conformation amino acids (Figure 6.2). The design was based on the unique architecture of the alternating isomers observed in some natural antibiotic peptides. The special design of the peptides

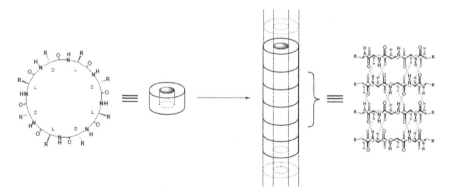

Figure 6.2: The formation of peptide nanotubes by the self-assembly of alternating L- and D-amino-acids. The peptide design resulted in the planar structure that allows the stacking of the peptides to form tubular hollow assemblies at the nano-scale. Courtesy of Dr. M. Reza Ghadiri. Reproduced from Bong *et al.* (2001), by permission of John Wiley and Sons.

resulted in flat ring-shaped subunits which are stacked together through intermolecular hydrogen bonds in a β-sheet conformation (Ghadiri *et al.*, 1993; 1994; Bong *et al.*, 2001). This conformation of a stacked β-sheet structure is similar to that of the nano-scale amyloid fibrils mentioned in Chapter 3.

The closed cycle and the alternating D- and L-conformations direct the side chains outwards from the ring and the backbone amides, approximately perpendicular to the ring plane. The self-assembly process and the geometry of the nanotubes were shown to be controlled by rationally changing the number of amino acids in the ring and the amino acid identity. The internal diameter of the nanotubes ranges between 0.7–0.8 nm and can be controlled by changing the number of the amino acids in the cyclic peptide sequence.

Follow-up studies by the same group demonstrated the ability to engineer the side chains of the peptide nano-structures (Bong *et al.*, 2001). This is especially important for the design of conductive nanotubes by the correct orientation of the organic systems which allow electron transfer in space through non-covalent systems (Horne *et al.*, 2005). This could lead to very important molecular nanoelectronic applications of these peptide nano-structures. Another practical application, already demonstrated for this class of peptide nanotubes, is their activity as antibacterial agents. This activity is achieved by the formation of nano-channels in the bacterial membrane by the nanotubes, which is similar to the effect of natural antimicrobial peptides on bacterial viability.

Another cyclic peptide reported to self-assemble into well-ordered tubular structures is the lanreotide octapeptide which is naturally synthesized as a growth hormone inhibitor and used for the treatment of a disease called acromegaly, a result of excess hormone secreted from the pituitary gland. The peptide folds into a β-hairpin (two beta strands connected by a short turn) which is stabilized by a disulfide bridge and intramolecular hydrogen bonds. Ultrastructural analysis revealed that the lanreotide peptide self-assembles into tubular structures with nanometric dimensions (tube diameter of 24.4 nm) in aqueous solution (Valery *et al.*, 2003). These nanotubes are suggested to self-assemble through the segregation of the aliphatic and aromatic residues which contribute to the conversion into β-sheet fibrils. The stacking of two hairpins forms the wall of the nanotube corresponding to a wall thickness of approximately 1.8 nm (Valery *et al.*, 2011). The self-assembly of the peptide leads to gel formation which is reversible, i.e., the tubes disassemble and lanreotide monomers are released upon dilution in water or physiological buffers. This property is exploited for the controlled delivery of the drug from gel implants, and it is actually an elegant example of the drug and self-assembling element being the same, with "just water" addition required for the formulation of the drug (see Somatuline® autogel from www.ipsen.com). The use of aromatic interactions with much smaller peptides, as simple as dipeptides, will be described further below.

6.4. Amphiphile and Surfactant-Like Peptide Building Blocks

Another direction for the assembly of ordered peptide structures at the nano-scale is to use the same physical principles which drive the formation of phospholipid membranes as described in Chapter 3. The design peptides use amphiphilic structures, just as the phospholipids, to form well-ordered structures at the nano-scale by hydrophobic interactions. Several groups have utilized this approach including the groups of Samuel Stupp, Hiroshi Matsui, and Shuguang Zhang (Figure 6.3).

The work of Stupp and co-workers utilizes amphiphile molecules composed of a long hydrophobic aliphatic tail and a hydrophilic peptide chain head, similar to the structure of phospholipid molecules (Hartgerink *et al.*, 2001; Silva *et al.*, 2004). Yet, the peptide headgroups allow the integration of biological information into the nano-assemblies. The suggested arrangement of the formed nano-fibril is of a cylindrical micelle in which the peptide part is perpendicular to the fiber axis, while the hydrophobic tail is placed in the fiber center and the hydrophilic head at the external part of the fiber. Researchers also use various modifications of the nano-structures such as cross-linking and mineralization. These were achieved by designing the peptide parts in such a way that they contain cysteine residues allowing thiol-metal interactions with the assemblies. By changing the nature of amino acids in the peptide part, further variations of these amphiphiles were designed and targeted for the binding of magnetic materials, contrast agents for MRI, or for cell adhesion and proliferation, etc. (Cui *et al.*, 2010).

Figure 6.3:   Formation of tubular and fibrillar structures by the self-assembly of short peptides by using hydrophobic or electrostatic interactions as driving force. Amphiphile picture reproduced courtesy of Dr. Hiroshi Matsui and with permission from Matsui, H., Pan, S., Gologan, B., and Jonas, S. H. (2000) Bolaamphiphile nanotube-templated metallized wires. *J. Phys. Chem. B*, **104**, 9576–9579. Copyright (2000) American Chemical Society (ACS). Surfactant-like picture reproduced courtesy of Dr. Shuguang Zhang and with permission from Vauthey, S., Santoso, S., Gong, H., Watson, N., and Zhang, S. (2002) Molecular self-assembly of surfactant-like peptides to form nanotubes and nanovesicles. *Proc. Natl. Acad. Sci. USA* **99**, 5355–5360. Copyright (2002) National Academy of Sciences, USA. Ionic complementarity picture reproduced courtesy of Dr. Shuguang Zhang and with permission from Holmes, T. C., de Lacalle, S., Su, X., Liu, G., Rich, A., and Zhang, S. (2000) Extensive neurite outgrowth and active synapse formation on self-assembling peptide scaffolds. *Proc. Natl. Acad. Sci. USA* **97**, 6728–6733. Copyright (2000) National Academy of Sciences, USA. The figure is modified from Reches and Gazit (2006) with permission from Bentham Science Publishers.

Peptide-based tubular structures can also self-assemble using linear peptides as demonstrated with a family of bolaamphiphile peptides by Matsui and co-workers (Banerjee *et al.*, 2003; Djalali *et al.*, 2003; Nuraje *et al.*, 2004). In these structures two hydrophilic peptides are conjugated through an aliphatic peptide linker (Figure 6.3). The driving force for the formation of these structures is the intermolecular association of the hydrophobic moieties in aqueous solution to form ordered structures similar to a micellization process. Tubular structures self-assembled by one of these peptides, bis(N-α-amido-glycylglycine)-1,7-heptane dicarboxylate were used as a template to form metal wires. These nanotubes were also immo-bilized to metallic surfaces via hydrogen bonds onto functionalized gold.

Later studies by Shuguang Zhang and co-workers demonstrated the ability to use native, rather than conjugated, peptides as building blocks to form ordered nano-scale structures (Holmes *et al.*, 2000; Kisiday *et al.*, 2002; Vauthey *et al.*, 2002). The design of the peptides was based on the use of the side chains and not external alkyl groups as the hydrophobic part, which allowed the design of the amphiphatic nature of the structures (Figure 6.3). The researchers designed a set of short peptides (7–8 amino acids) and used charged amino acid residues to build a hydrophilic head and aliphatic residues to construct a hydrophobic tail to form "surfactant-like" peptide molecules (Figure 6.3). Indeed these surfactant-like peptides undergo self-assembly to form nanotubes and nano-vesicles. The surfactant-like peptides were also used as mimicry of biological mem-branes to extract and stabilize membrane proteins.

These nano-scale-ordered peptides were also used to form macroscopic hydrogel assemblies. Hydrogel scaffolds made of peptides with altering hydrophilic and hydrophobic amino acids were used as a template for tissue-cell attachment, extensive neurite outgrowth, and formation of active nerve connections (Holmes *et al.*, 2000).

6.5. Charge Complementary as a Driving Force for Self-Assembly

An earlier approach by Shuguang Zhang and co-workers for the assem-bly of linear non-conjugated peptides was based not only on hydrophobic-ity, but mainly on self-complementary ionic peptides (Altman *et al.*, 2000; Figure 6.3). These linear peptides are highly (> 50 %) charged with opposite charges using alternately basic and acidic amino acids. The design was based on the molecular organization of a segment within the zuotin yeast protein. Moreover, the peptides are arranged to contain two distinct sur-faces, hydrophilic and hydrophobic. These peptides adopt β-sheet confor-mation and self-assemble into nanofibers. The self-assembly of the peptides was serendipitously discovered when they formed macroscopic membranes upon dissolving in phosphate-buffered saline (150 mM NaCl/10 mM sodium phosphate, pH 7.4, conditions used to mimic the biological milieus). These membranes were found to be resistant to proteolysis, detergents, and denaturants; furthermore, their cytocompatibility and lack of toxicity towards cell cultures opened the way for their use in applications. These nanofibers further form a hydrogel by changing the pH from acid to neutral, or by adding salt solutions in the concentration range used in cell growth media; the hydrogel allows extensive neurite outgrowth and therefore can be used as a scaffold for tissue engineering. Using this method Zhang opened the way for the use of hydrogels as scaffolds for cell attachment and proliferation of a variety of cell types (Gelain *et al.*, 2007; Hauser and Zhang, 2010; Horii *et al.*, 2007). We will further elaborate on these applications in Chapter 9.

Taking advantage of alternating hydrophobic and charged amino acids, peptides which are competent for controlled self-assembly can be *de novo* designed. An elegant example is the design of self-assembling β-hairpins from Schneider, Pochan, and colleagues. Two such alternating sequences connected by a sequence that enforces a turn can fold into an intramolecular hairpin once the charges of the positively charged residues are neutralized (Schneider *et al.*, 2002). Intramolecular hairpin folding is followed by intermolecular assembly through hydrogen bonds between hairpins and association between the hydrophobic presenting faces. In this way, β-structured fibrillar networks form, leading to rigid hydrogel formation. Assembly and hydrogel formation are reversible and can be modulated by lowering the pH below the pK of the charged residues. This results in disassembly due to charge repulsion and subsequently to unfolding of the individual hairpins. This system allows the introduction of responsiveness to temperature, pH or salt conditions through rational amino acid changes (Ozbas *et al.*, 2004).

Introducing responsiveness is very important for the use of these peptide networks as scaffolds for applications such as three-dimensional cell culture, controlled drug release, and tissue engineering. We will further elaborate on such applications in Chapter 9.

6.6. Conjugation of Peptides for Self-Assembly

Another approach for the self-assembly of peptide structures at the nano-scale is based on the bis-conjugation of short peptide elements (Figure 6.4). In a very interesting work by Sandeep Verma and co-workers,

Figure 6.4: Formation of fibrillar nano-structures by the design of peptide conjugates. Courtesy of Dr. Sandeep Verma. Reproduced from Madhavaiah and Verma (2004) with permission of the Royal Society of Chemistry. doi: 10.1039/B3167936

short peptide elements were conjugated in a symmetrical fashion to allow the formation of well-organized assemblies at the nano-scale (Madhavaiah and Verma, 2004; 2005). The conjugation of the short peptide elements allows the efficient assembly of structures which could be formed by the non-conjugated peptides. These include peptides that were derived from the prion protein which forms amyloids in the case of the deadly BSE syndrome (bovine spongiform encephalopathy or mad cow disease). The properties of the self-assembled amyloid nano-fibrils were already mentioned in Chapter 3 and will be described below. Clearly this self-organization of amyloid fibrils is a key process in biomolecular assembly which has ample technological applications.

6.7. Aromatic Interactions for the Formation of Nano-Structures

As mentioned above, hydrophobicity is one of the central driving forces in the formation of peptide-based nano-structures. This self-organization is achieved in a similar manner to the interaction between aliphatic moieties which lead to the formation of ordered structures. Another type of hydrophobic interaction which also provides order and directionality is the interaction between aromatic moieties.

The interaction between aromatic moieties is directional due to the exact and restricted geometry which is allowed between aromatic moieties (Hunter, 1993). As was mentioned in Chapter 3, this type of interaction was suggested to play a key role in the molecular recognition and self-assembly processes that lead to the formation of amyloid fibrils (Gazit, 2002a).

The use of specific aromatic interactions was demonstrated in the 1990s to form nano-scale assemblies (Aggeli *et al.*, 1997). Sheena Radford and co-workers designed a linear β-sheet peptide that contained aromatic moieties which mediated specific interactions between the moieties. As can be observed in Figure 6.5, the specific interactions between tryptophane and phenylalanine pairs resulted in the organization of the peptides that lead to the formation of well-ordered nano-tapes.

6.8. The Formation of Aromatic Dipeptide Nanotubes (ADNT)

As mentioned above, it has already been suggested and demonstrated that aromatic interactions play a central role in the molecular recognition and self-assembly processes that lead to the formation of nano-scale amyloid fibrils. It has been demonstrated by several groups that short aromatic peptides, as short as tetrapeptides, can form well-ordered amyloid nano-fibrils.

In the search for the shortest amyloidogenic peptide fragment, the diphenylalanine core motif of Alzheimer's disease, β-amyloid peptide, was

Figure 6.5: Formation of nano-tapes by the self-assembly of designed β-sheet aromatic peptides. Courtesy of Drs. Sheena Radford and Neville Boden. Reprinted with permission from Macmillan Publishers Ltd: [*Nature*] Aggeli, A., Bell, M., Boden, N., Keen, J. N., Knowles, P. F., McLeish, T. C., Pitkeathly, M., and Radford, S. E. (1997) Responsive gels formed by the spontaneous self-assembly of peptides into polymeric beta-sheet tapes. *Nature* **386**, 259–262. Copyright (1997).

studied (Figure 6.6). Quite surprisingly, this extremely simple peptide motif was found to form remarkably ordered nanotubes (Reches and Gazit, 2003; Song *et al.*, 2004). These hollow cylinders with an internal diameter of about 20 nm and external diameter that ranges from 80 to a few hundred nm are formed as discrete supramolecular assemblies with a very high persistence length. The peptides are formed by either L- or D-amino acid-based peptides which have indistinguishable ultrastructural properties but differ in their proteolytic stability. The use of these nanotubes for nanotech-nological applications has already been demonstrated (Reches and Gazit,

Figure 6.6: Formation of peptide nanotubes by the core recognition element of the β-amyloid polypeptide. From Reches, M. and Gazit, E. (2003) Casting metal nanowires within discrete self-assembled peptide nanotubes. *Science* **300**, 625–627. Reprinted with permission from AAAS.

2003; Song *et al.*, 2004; Yemini *et al.*, 2005a; 2005b) and will be further discussed in the following chapters.

The aromatic dipeptide nanotubes are very attractive building blocks for nanotechnology as they show remarkable thermal and chemical stability (Kol *et al.*, 2005). The peptide nanotubes also show extraordinary mechanical strength. With a Young's modulus of 20 GPa, they appear to be the most rigid bio-inspired nano-structures. The extreme mechanical strength of the peptide nanotubes is suggested as the result of an extensive array of interactions between the aromatic moieties of the building blocks. The mechanical properties of the aromatic polymers resemble those of the aromatic Nomex® and Kevlar® (Figure 6.7).

Figure 6.7: The chemical structure of the peptide nanotubes compared with some of the strongest known aromatic nylons which are used for technological applications.

These organic polymers are known to have very strong mechanical properties and are used for many applications. They are basically very similar to nylon, but have aromatic linkers instead of aliphatic ones. The main difference between these polymers and ADNT is the fact that the nanotubes are supramolecular assemblies formed by the self-association of simple building blocks in contrast to the high molecular weight polymers.

6.9. The Formation of Spherical Nano-Structures by Short Peptides

It was later revealed that diphenylglycine, a highly similar analogue and the simplest aromatic homo-dipeptide, does not form nanotubular structures but rather spherical nanometric assemblies (Figure 6.8; Reches and Gazit, 2004). The introduction of a thiol group into the diphenylalanine peptide also alters its assembly from tubular to spherical particles

Figure 6.8: The formation of spherical nanostructures by the assembly of modified short aromatic peptides. Reprinted with permission from Reches, M. and Gazit, E. (2004) Formation of closed-cage nanostructures by self-assembly of aromatic dipeptides. *Nano Lett.* **4**, 581–585. Copyright (2004) American Chemical Society.

similar to those formed by diphenylglycine. The formation of either nano-tubes or closed-cages by fundamentally similar peptides is consistent with a two-dimensional layer closure, as described in Chapter 2, both for carbon and inorganic nanotubes and their corresponding buckminster-fullerene and fullerene-like structures. These spherical nano-structures were recently found to have an extraordinary mechanical strength of up to 275 GPa and may have various applications in the reinforcement of poly-meric materials and biomaterials for implants and dental fillings, etc. (Adler-Abramovich *et al.*, 2010b).

6.10. Helical Peptide Building Blocks

Self-assembling systems, either natural or designed, are based mainly on β-structured building blocks. However, α-helical self-assembling systems were also designed and studied, mostly by the Conticello (Zimenkov *et al.*, 2004), Fairman (Wagner *et al.*, 2005) and Woolfson groups. Clever self-assembling systems can be designed by exploiting the rules which govern the folding of α-helical coiled-coils. Coiled-coils are formed when α-helices wind around each other — such structures are found in hair keratins and cytoskeletal proteins discussed earlier in Chapter 3. Coiled-coil sequences have a particular sequence signature of seven residues *abcdefg,* where positions *a* and *d* are occupied by hydrophobic residues, and *g* and *e* by charged residues — this is the so-called "heptad repeat". Residues *a* and *d* are buried at the interface between helices and the assembly is consolidated through electrostatic interactions between residues *e* and *g*. The Woolfson group designed 28 amino acid peptides that comprised alternating cationic and anionic heptad repeats. The anionic repeats were designed with negatively charged residues at positions *e* and *g*, whilst the cationic repeats were designed with positively charged residues at positions *e* and *g* (Ryadnov *et al.*, 2009). Alternating cationic and anionic repeats promote out-of-register electrostatic interactions at positions *e* and *f* and induce fibrillogenesis. The same group also pioneered the co-assembly of two peptide systems, called SAFs (self-assembling fiber peptides) (Pandya *et al.*, 2000). Co-assembly is promoted by designed "sticky ends" in the peptide sequences and consolidated by electrostatic interactions between oppositely charged heptad repeats. Based on this basic design, additional functionalities or morphologies (such as branches or kinks) can be introduced (Woolfson, 2010).

6.11. Peptide Nucleic Acids (PNA)

The majority of this chapter is devoted to DNA structures which utilize the remarkable specific recognition of nucleotides and to the peptides that serve as robust and very useful building blocks. A combination of both biomolecules is present in peptide nucleic acids (PNAs), a class of polymers with an amide backbone, as found in peptides, but with nucleic acid bases as the side chain (Nielsen, 1995). These molecules are synthesized using the conventional peptide chemistry techniques described above, but have much more advanced specific recognition properties as nucleic acids. Furthermore, the PNA polymers can form hetero-duplex assemblies with DNA or RNA and can be used for various molecular recognition applications (Briones and Moreno, 2012).

Chapter 7

Application of Biological Assemblies in Nanotechnology

In this chapter we will mainly consider bionanotechnology as defined in Chapter 1 (i.e., the use of biological and bio-inspired assemblies in the field of nanotechnology). Biological assemblies have indeed already been successfully used in various nanotechnological applications. One of the most advanced uses of biological assemblies is the formation of metallic wires at the nano-scale. For these applications various biomolecular assemblies were employed including DNA, proteins, and polypeptides. Some of the advancements in this direction include the use of molecular lithography and fabrication of coaxial nanowires. Such nano-structures may have actual uses that are not related to biology or medicine but to molecular electronics.

7.1. The Use of S-Layers for Nanolithography

The formation of the nano-scale-ordered S-layers was described in Chapter 3. These marvelous self-assembled nano-structures were demonstrated to be very useful for lithographic applications. Purified S-layer building blocks spontaneously reassemble into well-ordered two-dimensional crystals under *in vitro* conditions. This property was used by Uwe Sleytr and co-workers to demonstrate that it is possible to recrystallize S-layer subunits on various substrates which are suitable for nanofabrication, such as silicon or silicon oxide wafers (Figure 7.1). Other studies have shown the ability to arrange the layers in lipid membranes or at the air–water interface. S-layers have also been used as binding templates for well-organized arrangements of nanoparticles, such as semiconductors and metallic dots (Gyorvary *et al.*, 2004), and also for biomolecules such as enzymes and antibodies. This type

exposure with DUV
(ArF, 193nm)

lithographic mask

S-layer

silicon wafer

Figure 7.1: Schematic drawing of the patterning of an S-layer on a silicon wafer by DUV radiation using an ArF excimer laser. Courtesy of Dr. Uwe Sleytr. Reproduced from Pum, D., Neubauer, A., Gyorvary, E., Sara, M., and Sleytr, U. B. (2000) S-layer proteins as basic building blocks in a biomolecular construction kit. *Nanotechnol.* **11**, 100–107, by permission from IOP Publishing Ltd. doi:10.1088/0957-4484/11/2/310.

of assembly and molecular interaction allowed the application of the crystalline arrays as patterning media for nano-scale lithography (Figure 7.1).

It was demonstrated that it is possible to pattern S-layers using ultraviolet radiation (Figure 7.2). S-layers that were ordered on a silicon wafer are brought into direct contact with a photomask and exposed to ultraviolet irradiation. Such lithographic patterning of the layers, together with specific patterning of inorganic molecules and biomolecules could allow the fabrication of a lab-on-a-chip. Other suggested applications of S-layers include the fabrication of ultrafiltration membranes with well-defined molecular weight cutoffs and immobilization matrices for the binding of monolayers of functional molecules in a geometrically well-defined way. For a recent review on S-layer applications, see Ilk *et al.* (2011).

7.2. The Use of DNA for Fabrication of Conductive Nanowires

The usefulness of DNA as a building material at the nano-scale, elegantly demonstrated by Nadrian Seeman, was presented in Chapter 6. Yet,

Figure 7.2:   Scanning force microscopy image of a patterned S-layer on a silicon wafer. The bar represents a distance of 1000 nm. Courtesy of Dr. Uwe Sleytr. Reproduced from Pum, D., Neubauer, A., Gyorvary, E., Sara, M., and Sleytr, U. B. (2000) S-layer proteins as basic building blocks in a biomolecular construction kit. *Nanotechnol.* **11**, 100–107, by permission from IOP Publishing Ltd. doi:10.1088/0957-4484/11/2/310.

these remarkable DNA structures are rather inert. As we will discuss here, the specific properties of the DNA and its ability to specifically interact with various proteins have direct practical applications in nanotechnology. In this case DNA is being used as a nanowire with specific recognition information embedded.

One of the earliest attempts and most elegant demonstrations of the use of DNA as a bio-material for nanotechnology is the continuous work of Uri Sivan, Erez Braun, Yoav Eichen, and co-workers. At the first stages of their nanotechnological applications of DNA, the controlled metal coating of DNA molecules was demonstrated (Braun *et al.*, 1988). The researchers had used a process of silver deposition and enhancement to form uniform metallic wires on a double stranded DNA template. The wires were of a dimension of about 100 nm and were proven to have ohmic conductivity.

One of the great advantages of the DNA-based wires is the ability of the DNA to also serve as a carrier of address data that can help to direct the DNA strand into specific locations, which is a key step for the

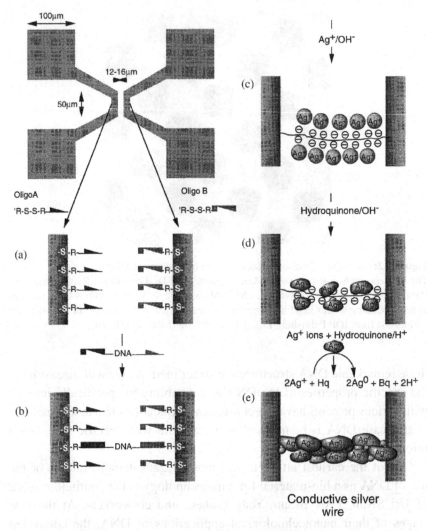

Figure 7.3:   The metallization of DNA oligomers to form conductive nanowires. Single-stranded DNA molecules were specifically targeted to surface-bound complementary DNA oligomers. The formed continuous DNA hybrid was further coated with silver to form conductive silver nano-wires. Courtesy of Dr. Erez Braun. Reprinted with permission from Macmillan Publishers Ltd: [*Nature*] Braun, E., Eichen, Y., Sivan, U., and Ben-Yoseph, G. (1998) DNA-templated assembly and electrode attachment of a conducting silver wire. *Nature* **391**, 775–778. Copyright (1998).

Photo Lithography   **Molecular Lithography**

Figure 7.4: Use of DNA-binding proteins for "molecular lithography". In photolithography, the silicon oxide surface is covered with a photoresist layer. The use of a mask leads to differential treatment of the photoresist and the etching of specific parts of the layer. In molecular lithography, the information encoded in the specific DNA sequence is the equivalent to that of a mask, and the DNA-binding protein serves as the equivalent of a resist. Reproduced from Gazit (2007), by permission of John Wiley and Sons.

achievement of self-assembled electronic circuits. Therefore, the same research groups went one step further and demonstrated the process of molecular lithography of a DNA molecule (Keren *et al.*, 2002). The researchers used RecA, a DNA protein which specifically binds to unique sequences on the DNA strand (Figure 7.4).

This design allowed the specific binding of the protein to the target DNA sequences and performed the metallization in such a way that parts of the DNA molecule were protected from the chemical process. Thus, the method allowed a sequence-specific and geometrically defined modification of the DNA molecule. The authors termed this process as molecular lithography. As was mentioned for conventional lithography in Chapter 2, the information encoded in the DNA molecules is equivalent to that of the masks used in conventional lithography, and the DNA-binding protein serves as the equivalent of a photoresist.

7.3. Amyloid Fibrils as Templates for Nanowire Fabrication

Protein and polypeptide fibrils are also very attractive templates for nano-scale molecular engineering (Hamada *et al.*, 2004). While proteins lack the simple recognition code which occurs with complementary nucleic acid strands it is important to note that proteins, and not nucleic acids, were the choice of evolution for structural elements in nature. Amyloid fibrils, as were described in Chapter 3, are very interesting due to their small diameter (7–10 nm) and remarkable physical and chemical stability. Amyloid fibrils are readily formed from quite simple building blocks. As was previously mentioned, it was shown that peptides as short as hexapeptides and pentapeptides can form typical amyloid fibrils (Tenidis *et al.*, 2000; Gazit, 2002b; Gilead and Gazit, 2005).

The ability of amyloid fibrils to serve as a template for the fabrication of nanomaterials was demonstrated with yeast prion proteins (Scheibel *et al.*, 2003). This protein could be synthesized on a large scale and readily assembled in the test tube. Such a prion protein was engineered to have an additional cysteine residue which is not present in the original protein. The exposed thiol group of this engineered protein served as a nucleation site for the deposition of the metal on the fibrils (Figure 7.5). As with the case of the DNA-based metallic nanowires, excellent conductivity could be observed upon the deposition of the metal wires between two electrodes.

The use of amyloid-forming peptides as templates for the fabrication of metal wires has very practical prospects as short peptides can form fibrils which are similar to those formed by the full length proteins and polypeptides. For example, metal binding by short octapeptides was achieved by introducing the cysteine residues that remain exposed out of the self-assembling peptide core to serve as nucleation sites for silver, gold, and platinum nanoparticles (Kasotakis *et al.*, 2009). Introducing exposed metal-binding residues can serve as a general strategy for metal binding even by shorter peptides. It was shown that even a modified dipeptide can form such typical amyloid fibrils (Reches and Gazit, 2005). This could allow the large-scale production of templates for the metallization and may provide a commercially viable solution for amyloid-based metallization.

Figure 7.5: Metal coating of the nano-scale protein amyloid fibrils. (a) Colloidal gold binds to specific thiols within the amyloid building blocks, followed by silver and gold enhancement to achieve metal coated fibrils as observed by various microscopy techniques ((b)–(d)). Courtesy of Dr. Thomas Scheibel. Reproduced from Scheibel, T., Parthasarathy, R., Sawicki, G., Lin, X. M., Jaeger, H., and Lindquist, S. L. (2003) Conducting nanowires built by controlled self-assembly of amyloid fibers and selective metal deposition. *Proc. Natl. Acad. Sci. USA* **100**, 4527–4532, with permission. Copyright (2003) National Academy of Sciences, USA.

7.4. Metallization of Actin Filaments by Chemical Modification

Other biological fibrils at the nano-scale which were mentioned previously in this book are the actin filaments. These are self-assembled fibrils of 7 nm diameter and have a very uniform organization. Furthermore, as the crystal structure of the actin monomers is known, new functionalities could be rationally engineered and introduced into the fibrillar system. Thus, these fibrils also serve as a very attractive platform for nano-scale engineering. One of the advantages of the actin filaments is the ability to control their polymerization and depolymerization by the presence of ATP nucleotides. It was indeed demonstrated by Itamar Willner and co-workers that re-polymerization of gold-coated actin filaments followed by the

Figure 7.6: Metal coating of actin fibrils. The fibrils are chemically reacted to bind gold nanoparticles, dialyzed, and re-polymerized with additional building blocks followed by gold enhancement. This results in continuous gold wires at the nano-scale. Courtesy of Dr. Itamar Willner. Reprinted with permission from Macmillan Publishers Ltd: [*Nature Materials*] Patolsky, F., Weizmann, Y., and Willner, I. (2004a) Actin-based metallic nanowires as bio-nanotransporters. *Nat. Mater.* **3**, 692–695. Copyright 2004.

catalytic enlargement of the nanoparticles allows the formation of conductive metal nanowires (Figure 7.6; Patolsky *et al.*, 2004a). Furthermore, the authors demonstrated the ATP-fueled motility of the actin-based wires on a myosin interface. Taken together, the actin-based molecular platform could combine selective metallization but also mechanical properties at the nano-scale, forming a genuine biomolecular nanoelectromechanical (BioMEMS) system.

Recombinant DNA technology offers the possibility of constructing multi-component biomolecules through the combination of assembly and binding motifs. Recently, a prokaryotic tubulin analog, FtsZ (filamentous temperature-sensitive protein) was bacterially expressed in the same plasmid with sequences encoding either silver-reducing or gold-binding peptide motifs previously identified by phage display (see Section 7.6). The resulting proteins combine the GTP-driven polymerization with metal-binding ability (Ostrov and Gazit, 2010).

7.5. The Use of Aromatic Peptide Nanotubes

Another group of bio-inspired materials that were used for the fabrication of metallic nanowires are aromatic dipeptide nanotubes. These supramolecular assemblies are hollow with an inner diameter of a few tens of nanometers. In the case of the tubes, the preferential entrance of metal ions into the lumen of the tubes allowed the formation of wires within the tubes rather than coating the outside of the biomolecule (Figure 7.6; Reches and Gazit, 2003). The use of biological proteolytic enzymes then allowed the degradation of the peptide coating and enabled us to obtain silver wires of a diameter of only 20 nm. This size of metal wire is smaller than can be achieved by conventional lithography. The remarkable rigidity of the nanotubes allowed us to obtain elongated nanowires with very high persistence length (Figure 7.7).

As with the other biological materials described above, the peptide nanotubes could also be coated with an outer metallic layer. The

Figure 7.7: Formation of silver nanowires with peptide nanotubes templates. Ionic silver is reduced to metallic silver within the tube lumen. The peptide envelope is then removed by the use of enzymatic degradation. From Reches, M. and Gazit, E. (2003) Casting metal nanowires within discrete self-assembled peptide nanotubes. *Science* **300**, 625–627. Reprinted with permission from AAAS.

combination of the deposition of metal within the peptide tube but also in the outer layer allows the fabrication of coaxial metal wires at the nano-scale (Carny *et al.*, 2006). Such coaxial wires should have several applications in molecular electronics.

7.6. Bacteriophages as Novel Biomaterials

Another very interesting building block for nanotechnology is the bacteriophage, a virus that infects bacteria. In a pioneering work, Angela M. Belcher and co-workers were able to engineer phage particles for nano-technology applications. The great advantage of the phage particles is their ability to express specific proteins on their surface in multiple copies. The utilization of these properties for the selection of high-affinity peptides from a library was described in Chapter 5.

Belcher and co-workers described the use of short peptides which were selected for their high affinity to inorganic material in order to fabricate magnetic, semiconductive and conductive nanowires (S. W. Lee *et al.*, 2002; Mao *et al.*, 2004). Short peptides with affinity for various metals and semiconductors were displayed at the surface of coat proteins of the phage and were used for the fabrication of more complex assemblies with nano-scale order. Further work by this group demonstrated the usefulness of the phage-based nano-ordered strategy for the design and fabrication of lithium-ion battery electrodes (Nam *et al.*, 2006).

Short peptides selected with phage display techniques for binding to inorganic materials are versatile tools which can either be used by themselves, or in conjugation with other macromolecular assemblies or building blocks, for example, DNA, proteins, and peptides. Nowadays, a large spectrum of peptides exists, selected for specific binding to noble metals, oxides, semiconductors, and minerals such as hydroxyapatite, calcite etc. The groups of Mehmet Sarikaya and Candan Tamerler coined the term GEPIs for "genetically engineered peptides for inorganics" to designate peptides selected through combinatorial methods and pioneered their use for directed assembly, linking, and positioning of inorganic nanoparticles and conjugated biomolecules (Tamerler *et al.*, 2010). These peptide sequences can also be recombinantly coexpressed with proteins (Kacar *et al.*, 2009), or incorporated in self-assembling peptide sequences

(Gungormus *et al.*, 2010), to produce multifunctional materials for various applications. More examples of macromolecular assemblies which have recently been extensively investigated as macromolecular scaffolds for inorganic materials are filamentous viruses such as TMV, spherical viruses, and bacterial flagellae. The surface of the TMV virion is rich in both negatively and positively charged residues and can be used for the templating of inorganic nanoparticles, such as metals and semiconductors etc., through electrostatic interactions (Dujardin *et al.*, 2003; Lee *et al.*, 2006). Furthermore, insertion of cysteine residues, through genetic engineering, on the TMV surface does not affect the assembly and stability of the virus. These genetically modified scaffolds were used for the deposition of gold, silver, and palladium nanoparticles and the creation of metallic biocomposite nanowires (Lee *et al.*, 2005).

Icosahedral viruses, devoid of their nucleic acid, can be used as templates and nano-containers ("viral protein cages") for nanomaterial synthesis. These approaches were pioneered by Trevor Douglas and Mark Young (Douglas *et al.*, 2002; Douglas, 2003). Bogdan Dragnea recently demonstrated that gold nanoparticles can mimic the charge effects of DNA, acting as templates for the organization of positively charged viral capsid proteins, resulting in the formation of "viral-like particles" (VLPs), (Chen *et al.*, 2006). Both viral cages and VLPs may have important applications in imaging, drug delivery, enzymic catalysis or as single enzyme nanoreactors etc. (Aniagyei *et al.*, 2008).

The bacterial flagellum that we described as a molecular motor in Chapter 3 is composed of thousands of self-assembling subunits of the protein flaggelin. Solvent-exposed loops in the protein can be used, through genetic engineering, for the insertion of sequences targeted for templating inorganic materials. Histidine (a metal-binding amino acid) sequences were used for the templating of gold, copper, cobalt, palladium, cadmium nanoparticles, and cadmium telluride quantum dots (Kumara *et al.*, 2007a; 2007b).

7.7. The Use of Peptide Templates for Biomineralization

Although most of the building blocks in biology are based on organic, carbon-dominated building blocks such as proteins, nucleic acids, polysaccharides, and phospholipids, the role of inorganic materials could not be ignored. The physical strength of skeletal tissues, bones, and teeth is based on the organization of inorganic materials. The most notable mineral is, of course, calcium in its different forms. Consequently, calcium uptake and organization has a central role in human health. Human disorders such as osteoporosis are associated with abnormal accumulation and organization of calcium in human bone. Yet, various organisms use other minerals such as silica as will be discussed in this chapter.

Bones clearly represent the most predominantly inorganic biological tissue. Bone contains about 30% organic material mostly in the form of collagen fibrils which provides the bone with strength and flexibility. These are the same collagen protein fibrils which have a central role in other tissues such as skin and tendons, as were mentioned in Chapter 3. The remaining 70% of bone tissue is made up of inorganic materials, the calcium portion of which contains hydroxyapatite mineral, which is composed of various forms of calcium including calcium phosphate, calcium carbonate, calcium fluoride, calcium hydroxide, and citrate. Most of the calcium in the bones exists in crystalline rods with a thickness of 1–2 nm, width of 2–4 nm, and length of 20–40 nm.

Another important animal tissue which includes mostly inorganic material is the dental structure. The dentine layer of the tooth contains about 70% inorganic material, while the harder outer enamel coating contains about 98% inorganic material. As in the case of bone, the main inorganic constituent of the dental tissue is a calcium-based hydroxyapatite mineral. In most cases, proteins direct and organize the deposition of calcium inorganic phases in an epitaxial manner. This is mediated through acid amino acid sequences which serve as nucleation sites for calcium ions (Addadi and Weiner, 1992). Producing biomimetic materials targeted for hard tissue regeneration is based on the exploitation of these interaction principles. However, extraction and purification of the entire natural proteins involved in these processes stumbles into considerable technical difficulties. Many alternative approaches have been recently developed involving peptide amphiphiles (Hartgerink *et al.*, 2001), self-assembling peptides (Kirkham *et al.*, 2007), and naturally fibrous proteins such as silk (Bhumiratana *et al.*, 2011). These templates mostly contain acid residues targeted for calcium nucleation, or GEPIs selected for hydroxyapatite binding (Gungormus *et al.*, 2010).

7.8. Production of Inorganic Composite Nanomaterials

Biological molecules serve in many cases as templates for the organization of macroscopic inorganic matter. This process is known as biomineralization (Mann and Weiner, 1999). The formation of hard tissues in organisms such as those mentioned above (bone, teeth, and shells) is facilitated by the crystallization of inorganic minerals such as calcium carbonate using a biopolymeric template. The formed biocomposites are significantly different from the crystals which are formed by the inorganic material by itself with no template. A classical example is the formation of mother-of-pearl in mollusks. The shell is a remarkable composite material, made up from alternating layers of calcium carbonate in the form of aragonite and protein/polysaccharide (chitin) layers. This "brick-and-mortar architecture" of 95 % inorganic matter/5 % organic matter confers on the shells their extraordinary resistance to fracture (3,000 times more than aragonite alone) (Espinosa *et al.*, 2009; Fratzl and Weinkamer, 2007). Actually, the crystals may be "molded" into complicated macroscopic structures that have non-faceted crystal surfaces. All of this has, of course, been performed at a physiological temperature and pressure.

While calcium carbonate is the major interest in biomineralization related to human inorganic structures, it is worth mentioning that biogenic oxides and especially silica are one of the most investigated minerals in nature. The Earth's crust is composed of almost 30 % silicon, usually in its stable form of silicon dioxide SiO_2 or metal silicates. Silica biomineralization is very common in marine organisms and allows the formation of remarkable patterning of silica at the nano-scale. One of the most vivid examples is that of diatoms, micron-scale unicellular algae. These tiny creatures show astonishing organization of silica in their outer shells which have micron-scale organization (Perry and Keeling-Tucker, 2000). These structures are compatible with silica structures formed by lithography or at a high temperature and pressure.

The formation of silica in diatoms is templated by an organic matrix which consists of a family of proteins called silaffins. Following the difficult but successful extraction of silaffin-1, it was found that the sequence contains repeats with many post-translationally modified, positively charged amino acids (Kroger *et al.*, 1999). The extracted protein

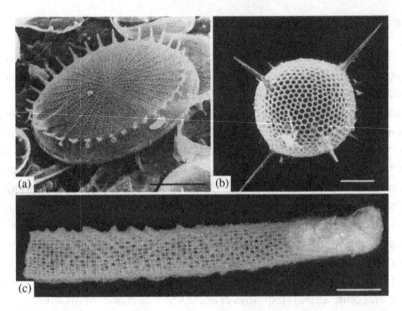

Figure 7.8: Marine organisms formed by directed organization of silica minerals. (a) diatom, scale bar = 5 μm, (b) radiolarian, scale bar = 20 μm, (c) sponge, *Euplectella* Owen, scale bar = 2,5 cm. Courtesy of Dr. Carole Perry. With kind permission from Springer Science+Businesss Media: *J. Biol. Inorg. Chem.*, **5**, 2000, 537, Perry, C. C. and Keeling-Tucker, T., Figure 1.

exhibits silica precipitation activity *in vitro* (condensating of an orthosilicic acid precursor) even at around pH 4.

Another class of marine organisms which biofabricate silica are orange puffball sponges. Their silica spicules are organized around an organic filament consisting of proteins called silicateins (Shimizu *et al.*, 1998). Natural and recombinant silicatein subunits have been found to catalyze the formation of biosilica from various silica precursors such as tetraethyl orthosilicate (TEOS) (Cha *et al.*, 1999). Pioneering work by the group of Daniel Morse showed that silicatein displays homology to proteolytic enzymes which contain a strongly nucleophilic hydroxyl amino acid (serine) in their active site (Shimizu *et al.*, 1998). This strongly nucleophilic residue initiates the hydrolysis of silica precursors followed by polycondensation. Another intricate architecture is used in the spicules of deep-sea sponges like the "Venus's flower basket" pictured in Figure 7.8c. These spicules are layered composite silica fibers organized around a central organic filament, resulting in a "core" with a high refractive index and a "cladding" with low refractive index (Aizenberg *et al.*, 2005). As a result, they act as optical waveguides with remarkable similarities to the optical fibers used in telecommunications (Sundar *et al.*, 2003; Aizenberg *et al.*, 2004).

7.9. The Utilization of Biomineralization in Nanotechnology

There is a great interest in the utilization of biomineralization in nano-technology. The ability to form complex inorganic structures, such as artificial bones and teeth, using biological templates which will direct inorganic organization may change the face of modern medicine. As we previously mentioned, extraction and purification of all the proteins involved is quite a technical challenge, therefore many *in vitro* approaches employ self-assembling building blocks endowed with templating activity. Knowledge of the mechanisms of biomineralization can lead to the nano-fabrication of artificial building blocks which emulate the original biotemplating behavior. Many studies are focused on examining the various bioorganic templates that will allow the crystallization of macroscopic structures.

Other work is directed toward using the diatom principles for the fabrication of silicon at the nano-scale. This is especially intriguing as it may allow the parallel fabrication of silicon-based structures compared with the serial fabrication by lithographic methods (Brott *et al.*, 2001). One example of such an approach is the use of a peptide fragment, of the previously mentioned silaffin-1 internal repeats protein, which mediates silica organization. The peptide fragment, which comprises the amino acid sequence of one repeat unit, can direct and affect the morphology of silica organization at near neutral pH (Naik *et al.*, 2003). Designer self-assembling peptides can be targeted for silica deposition through the introduction of positively charged residues which attract negatively charged silica precursors. Such examples include the β-hairpin (Altunbas *et al.*, 2010; Pouget *et al.*, 2007) or α-helical (Banwell *et al.*, 2009) peptides described in Chapter 6. Silicatein filaments are able to template not only silica, but also non-biogenic oxides such as titanium dioxide and gallium oxide at ambient temperatures and near neutral pH (Brutchey and Morse, 2008; Kisailus *et al.*, 2005; Tahir *et al.*, 2005). Serine-containing peptides which mimic the silicatein mechanism can template silica, titanium oxide, and germanium oxide nanoparticles (Dickerson *et al.*, 2004; Zhao *et al.*, 2012). Such biotemplated oxides can have numerous applications in hydrogen storage, catalysis, or drug delivery and controlled release applications (Patwardhan, 2011).

Chapter 8

Medical and Other Applications
of Bionanotechnology

One of the key future directions for nanobiotechnology and bionanotechnology is their medical use. As was mentioned briefly in the previous chapters, the use of nano-structures has already proven to be very useful in various applications, including drug delivery, ultrasensitive sensors, and the development of diagnostic tools. In this chapter we will first describe the application of nano-structures, biological and non-biological, as well as nanotechnology tools and techniques for various medical applications. The applications which will be described in this chapter are genuine and concrete, and some of them are to be employed in the near future. In Chapter 9, we will describe some of the more futuristic applications of nano-science and nanotechnology in years to come such as tissue engineering and even *in situ* cellular DNA manipulation to treat genetic defects. While medical and human treatment applications represent a major part of these activities, it is worth remembering that other applications are of high importance. This includes the use of nanobiotechnology and bionanotechnology in agriculture, water technology, cosmetics, and other applications which will be mentioned in the second part of the chapter.

8.1. The Use of Drug Nanocrystals for Improved Application

One of the most straightforward directions for nanotechnology to improve the effect of pharmaceutical products is to form nanocrystals of the desired drug. This is in contrast to the unordered powder or solidified powder as commonly used. The size of the nanocrystals is larger than that described for inorganic crystals at the nano-scale and is in the order of 200–500 nm. The nanocrystals are then administered as a suspension in aqueous solution.

This method offers various advantages over simple drug formulations as it offers much better solubility for hydrophobic drugs which are not water-soluble. It improves the bioavailability of the drug for absorption in the digestive track. Finally, it improves the stability of the drug to biological degradation in the body, as well as chemical and physical degradation which is reflected by a longer shelf life.

Several nanodrug formulations have been approved by the FDA in the last few years. One of the early nanocrystal drugs approved by the FDA is the immunosuppressant Rapamune® of Wyeth Pharmaceuticals. The approved formulation in 2000 significantly improved the availability and pharmacokinetics of the drug. Current attempts are being made in the nano-formulation of large peptide drugs such as insulin and other hormones for oral administration.

8.2. The Use of Nano-Containers for Drug Delivery

A more complex way of using nanotechnology for drug delivery is the use of heterologous nano-containers. As was briefly mentioned in our earlier discussion on the molecular basis of lipid vesicle self-assembly, one of the earliest applications of liposomes is the delivery of drugs to specific organs (Figure 8.1). The liposomes have many advantages due to their relative stability and ability to retain biological molecules with a low rate of leakage. Moreover, they are composed of natural biomolecules and thus are recognized as "self" material by the human body. Their chemical functionality allows their decoration with various biological and chemical molecules for specific targeting of the vesicles by high affinity to specific ligands or receptors.

Such high affinity is crucial for the delivery of highly toxic drugs such as chemotherapy agents. The specific targeting of such liposomes to the targeted tissue or organ allows us to use larger amounts of chemotherapy by reducing the overall side effects due to minimal exposure of the healthy tissue to the drug.

The encapsulation of the drug within the nano-container also affects the absorption, distribution, and metabolism of the drug and can result in better treatment protocols which are friendlier to the patient.

Figure 8.1: The use of phospholipid liposomes for drug delivery applications. Liposomes as closed-caged nano-containers can serve in various delivery applications. The biocompatibility of the liposomes and ability to decorate them with biological and chemical recognition elements allows their targeting to specific locations within the body. The liposomes can be used to deliver not only drugs but also genetic material for gene therapy applications.

The liposomes can be used not only for the delivery of drugs but also for the delivery of other materials such as DNA. This represents the applications of liposome technology for gene therapy, as normal genes can be transferred to cells carrying mutated, non-functional ones. This may be useful for various genetic diseases such as cystic fibrosis in which the newborn carries a mutated gene that does not allow a normal function. This could also be applicable for tumor cells which have mutated tumor suppressor genes as a result of a somatic mutation due to the exposure to carcinogens. Liposomes, or other nano-containers which could be decorated with specific recognition elements, could be used as an alternative to the current application of viral vectors to deliver the genes of interest. The use of the viral vectors is problematic due to various side effects resulting from the viral integration into the patient genome. Thus, a biologically inert delivery system may offer various advantages. In the case of gene delivery applications, cationic lipids rather than the naturally anionic lipids are used. These positively charged phospholipids form lipid vesicles by exactly the same driving force as the natural phospholipids (Hart, 2005). Yet, the net positive charge allows the high affinity interaction with the polyanionic negatively-charged DNA.

While the discussion above was devoted mainly to phospholipids, other nano-scale biocompatible containers could be used for various delivery applications as described for the liposomes. These include biomolecular-based vehicles such as the peptide nano-spheres and nano-vesicles mentioned in Chapter 6, as well as other organic and even inorganic structures which could allow the encapsulation of the cargo on the one hand and its desired release at the target on the other. Amongst these vehicles, amphiphilic block copolymers and self-assembling proteins and peptides are mostly used, due to their ability to self-assemble into vesicles, micelles, and hydrogels. Vesicles are hollow lamellar (either unilamellar or multilamellar) structures with an aqueous interior, while micelles comprise a hydrophobic core and an aqueous shell. Hydrogels are fibrillar non-covalently linked networks which can entrap water at values up to 99 %. Many commercially available containers made of block copolymers, proteins, and peptides are used nowadays for controlled delivery of anticancer drugs, antifungal, and antimicrobial small molecules (Branco and Schneider, 2009). Moreover, small molecules, growth factors, proteins, and entire cells can be encapsulated in hydrogels, and injected *in situ* (Phillips *et al.*, 2010). Hydrogel forming peptides designed by the Shuguang Zhang group, described in Chapter 6, are commercially available now under the name Puramatrix™ (www.puramatrix.com). These and other hydrogel forming self-assembling peptides reviewed in Chapter 6 are increasingly used as drug delivery containers that gel *in situ*. (Loo *et al.*, 2012). Of special interest are those containers which can reversibly self-assemble depending on external stimuli, such as temperature, pH or even shear stress. This gives the opportunity to encapsulate the desired "cargo" before delivery and release it *in situ* through triggered disassembly of the container. An elegant demonstration of triggered assembly-disassembly was made with the designer β-hairpin peptides from the Schneider and Pochan groups that we also saw in Chapter 6. These peptides can be designed to undergo triggered assembly and hydrogelation upon addition of cell culture media directly in a syringe container; cells can be encapsulated under these conditions. The shear stress created by depressing the syringe plunger induces thinning of the hydrogel, which flows and can be delivered to the desired site where it immediately reforms (Haines-Butterick *et al.*, 2007). As of 2012, many patents have appeared on the use of self-assembling peptides in drug delivery and tissue engineering (Kumar *et al.*, 2011).

8.3. The Use of Inorganic Nanowires for Biological Detection

Other important tools in the development of ultra-sensitive devices are semiconductor nanowires, most importantly silicon nanowires. Charles M. Lieber and co-workers demonstrated a very sensitive use of silicon nanowires for biological applications (Patolsky *et al.*, 2004b; Zheng *et al.*, 2005; Wang *et al.*, 2005). These one-dimensional nano-objects are modified with high-affinity antibodies (see Chapter 5) and their interaction could be detected at very high sensitivity using nanowire field effect transistors (Figure 8.2). The conductivity of the nanowires is so sensitive to the binding of the biological molecules that even the binding of a single viral particle could be detected and recorded (Patolsky *et al.*, 2004b). Such sensitivity has immense importance for many applications including early detection of various diseases, environmental, and homeland security detection of biological and chemical agents, and the modulation of various nano-devices and nano-machines.

Figure 8.2:   The use of silicon nanowires for the detection of biological interactions. The binding of charged ligands affects the current of either p-type or n-type silicon nanowires. The level of interaction could be monitored in real-time to provide information not only on the amount of ligands but also on the kinetics of the association and dissociation.

In a later study, the authors demonstrated the electrical detection of biomarkers using multiplexed nanowire sensor arrays (Zheng *et al.*, 2005). Such a device allows the simultaneous monitoring of the interaction of a large number of ligands. As in the case of viral detection, the sensitivity was very high and subpicogram concentrations of a biological marker could be detected by the array. The ability to monitor the electric signal as a function of time also allows the determination of the kinetics of the association and dissociation of the molecules. Thus, the nanowire multiarray serves as an alternative to the surface plasmon resonance (SPR) methods as mentioned in Chapter 4. As in the case of SPR the nanowires allow the detection without the use of any external labeling. Yet, much higher sensitivity could be achieved. Nevertheless, it should be stressed that since the semiconductor nanowires are based on the gating of a transistor, the effect occurs only through the binding of charged ligands which can either increase or decrease the electrical current depending on the type of silicon nanowires. In the case of the p-type nanowire (silicon that contains trivalent impurities such as boron or aluminum which are missing an electron in their outer electron shell), the conductance should decrease when the surface charge of the ligand is positive and increase when the surface charge is negative. The opposite is true for n-type silicon which contains atoms such as arsenic that contain an unpaired electron.

Carbon nanotubes, due to their stability, electronic properties, and the possibility of being chemically modified, have also attracted lots of interest for their use in sensing. Due to their porous character and high aspect ratio, they improve the surface coverage of electrodes and can accumulate analytes from the monitored solution, increasing the sensitivity in electrochemical sensing (Balasubramanian and Burghard, 2006). Self-assembling peptides and nanotubes can be used instead, resulting in an increased sensitivity than that of carbon nanotubes (Adler-Abramovich *et al.*, 2010a; Yemini *et al.*, 2005a; 2005b). Therefore, they can offer a biological counterpart to carbon nanotubes, since they can be produced in ambient temperatures and aqueous environments. Peptide nanotubes can also assume the role of both the recognition and sensing elements in impedimetric sensor chips. Peptide nanotubes modified with an antivirus antibody can be positioned by dielectrophoresis between electrodes; binding of the virus particle increases the impedance and the event can be detected by measuring the capacitance variation (de la Rica *et al.*, 2008).

Exploiting the optical properties of nanoparticles for biosensing and bioassays is another domain which has shown an exponential increase in the last 15 years (Aili and Stevens, 2010). Suspensions of spherical gold particles with nanometer-sized diameters display a variety of intense colors. This is due to the phenomenon of SPR mentioned in Chapter 4. When the effect is localized at the surface of the nanometer-sized particles, it is called localized surface plasmon resonance (LSPR). It results in certain portions of the visible light being reflected, yielding, for example, a bright red color for gold nanoparticles with a diameter of around 30 nm. Of note, this property has been used since antiquity to produce the bright red colors in glassmaking (Freestone *et al.*, 2007); as nanoparticles get larger in size, the shifting of the reflected wavelength results in a color change visible to the naked eye, for example, a purple color for particles around 60 nm. This property change lies at the basis of the development of optical bioassays, where the analyte induces the assembly or the disassembly of particles, resulting in a color readout. For optimal results, small analytes are required compared with the size of nanoparticles; therefore, oligonucleotides and peptides are ideal. Peptide-functionalized gold nanoparticles are used for enzymic bioassays of very important enzymes such as proteases, kinases, and phosphatases. The basis of these assays lies in the aggregation or disaggregation of the particles induced by the enzyme action on the immobilized peptide (Stevens and Mecklenburg, 2012).

8.4. The Use of Soft Lithography for Biotechnology

The use of conventional lithography, as mentioned in Chapter 2, is one of the cornerstones of the modern microelectronic industry. Another type of fabrication of nanomaterials on surfaces is known as soft lithography or microcontact printing. This technique was developed by George M. Whitesides and co-workers, and has central applications in nanotechnology in general and nanobiotechnology in particular (Whitesides *et al.*, 2001; Shim *et al.*, 2003). The technique of soft lithography is based on the use of a micro-patterned stamp which is made of a poly(dimethylsiloxane) (PDMS). The elastic and transparent PDMS stamp is patterned using a fabricated master mold. The stamp is transparent not only to visible light but also to ultraviolet radiation down to 240 nm.

The PDMS stamp by itself is very useful for various biological applications. The physical properties of the stamp as mentioned above together with its excellent chemical resistance, thermal stability, and biocompatibility make it an excellent system to pattern microfluidic devices with patterned water-filled microchannels. Such settings allow the probing of the properties of single cells under various experimental conditions. The response of cells and unicellular organisms to varied external signals, their changes under various chemical and biological conditions, their chemotaxis (response to the gradient of chemical signals such as the attraction of the sperm to the egg), their cytometry (the chemical composition of the cells), and their differentiation could be studied at the single cell level (Li Jeon *et al.*, 2002; Wang and Ho, 2004; Wu *et al.*, 2004).

Another very interesting use of soft lithography is its application for the printing of organic molecules including protein molecules. Under these conditions the stamp is inked with a solution containing the organic molecules, the stamp is then rinsed and dried, then follows the printing of the molecules on the surface. Such applications allowed the printing of various peptides and proteins into nano-structured patterns (Kane *et al.*, 1999; Foley *et al.*, 2005). Such organization is useful for applications such as the fabrication of biosensors, the formation of protein and DNA arrays, and the organization of biological signaling molecules for tissue engineering (as will be further elaborated in Chapter 9).

Given the exponential increase of reports concerning applications of peptide-based biomaterials in the last decade, novel methods for their controlled assembly, positioning, and integration into devices are being developed. Aromatic dipeptide nanotubes can form vertical "nanoforests" upon evaporation from very volatile fluorinated alcohols on siliconized glass surfaces (Reches and Gazit, 2006b). Chemical vapor deposition methods were also developed for the diphenylalanine nanotube powders described above. Due to the inherent volatility of aromatic moieties, when heated on a heating stage at 200 °C, the peptide molecules evaporate and subsequently condense on a substrate surface placed above the heating source, forming hollow nanotubes perpendicularly oriented to the substrate surface. The technique is applicable to a variety of substrates, such as glass, carbon, gold, and silicon dioxide (Adler-Abramovich *et al.*, 2009). We will further discuss integration of bottom-up assembly methods with traditional top-down techniques in Chapter 9.

Direct laser writing of biological molecules also gained increasing interest in the last decade. The big advantage of the laser techniques is the possibility of direct writing without the use of a mask, mold or stamp, and their compatibility with aqueous solutions. For example, femtosecond laser non-linear lithography is based on the phenomenon of two-photon polymerization. Tight focusing of a beam of an ultrafast infrared laser into the volume of a photosensitive material can initiate the polymerization process by two-photon absorption within the focal region. Thus, three-dimensional structures can be fabricated by moving the laser focus three-dimensionally through the photosensitive material (Drakakis *et al.*, 2006). A variety of biological molecules can be subsequently positioned on these structures through thiol chemistry, biotin–avidin interactions, etc. The precise three-dimensional patterning of self-assembled peptide fibrils has recently been demonstrated on three-dimensional micro-structures using these techniques (Dinca *et al.*, 2008).

8.5 Contrast Agents by Nanomagnetic Materials

Another important application, which should enjoy very important advancement due to nanotechnology developments, is the field of MRI contrast agents. MRI is an excellent imaging method in terms of safety and the ability for very accurate three-dimensional tomography. Unlike X-ray-based tomography techniques such as computerized tomography (CT) which is based on powerful X-ray electromagnetic radiation that can be harmful, the MRI techniques are based on the differential interaction of various biological entities with an intense magnetic field. This represents a much safer application with a long monitoring time. Indeed, MRI techniques are being used to follow dynamic processes within the body. Techniques such as functional MRI (fMRI) allows the following of very complex processes, such as cognition, by the continuous monitoring of brain function upon the completion of various tasks. Yet, MRI, like all magnetic resonance techniques, is not very sensitive.

As this is a magnetic resonance technique, the imaging agents for MRI are ferromagnetic entities. This may involve iron-based compounds, including oxides just like the magnetic material that we have on our computer hard disks, or metals such gadolinium. The application of the ferromagnetic metals by themselves is limited due to questions of availability and safety and they are used as part of organic-based complexes. Nanoscale vehicles can allow the encapsulation of many ferromagnetic particles in dense packing to significantly enhance the sensitivity of the technique. Viral cages and peptide amphiphiles have been used for proof-of-principle (Bull *et al.*, 2005; Liepold *et al.*, 2009). Furthermore, as with drug delivery, these agents can be specifically modified to allow precise targeting of the nano-vesicles. Targeting of the nano-carriers to specific disease-related receptors can allow the detection of events such as cancer. The possibility of combining vehicles for targeting diseased tissues followed by the delivery of therapeutic agents along with diagnostic agents recently gave rise to the concept of "theranostics" (from "therapeutics" and "diagnostics") (Caldorera-Moore *et al.*, 2011).

8.6. Nanoagriculture

While most of the discussion regarding the utilization of nanotechnology is directed towards medical applications, it should be remembered that agriculture is also a very large and important field with significant economic and social implications. Agriculture provides the food that we eat and the wood for furniture and construction. Furthermore, with the constant rising price of oil and natural gas, and the depletion of the world reserves, in the future it might also be a source of energy as well as a source of starting materials for the chemical industry. Nanotechnology could actually offer many important diagnostic and therapeutic tools, initially directed for human use, to agriculture. This is of course trivial in the case of animal science, as many of the therapeutic and diagnostic methods developed for human beings could be directly applied to domesticated animals. Just as vaccination and the use of antibiotics revolutionized animal agricultural practice, so should future nanotechnological applications. Nanotechnology could also provide major advancement in plant growing agriculture. It should be noted that over the years, plant agriculture has become a very advanced scientific discipline and the production of agricultural products per given area is constantly increasing. The application of nanotechnology to this field includes the slow release of nutritional elements and minerals for nano-scale delivery systems. These systems could be designed in a way that would not just release the compounds in a constant pre-designed way, but could be a nano-scale machine that will detect the exact situation of the plant and its external surroundings to provide the best optimized growth conditions.

8.7. Water Technology and Nanotechnology

Water technologies are quickly becoming a very important part of 21st century industry. Water technology includes various aspects of water desalination and treatment as well as the monitoring of water quality. The need for better technologies for the water industry is not only limited to arid areas with limited water supply, but also to large industrial and urban areas that have to take care of the treatment of increasing volumes of sewage. Major companies such as General Electric and others have invested considerable effort to position themselves in this fast growing field (see: http://www.gewater.com/).

The water technology field can benefit from nanotechnological applications. Most water treatment facilities are based on the use of filters with nano-scale pores and inherent selectivity for water compared with salt and pollutants. The design of new membranes that have better ultra-filtration performance, should lead both to the improvement of the quality as well as to the lowering of the cost of the desalination and water treatment. Bionanotechnology could have a special role in these efforts. As the materials to form the membrane should be biocompatible, hydrophilic, and non-toxic, biological assemblies such as nano-scale nanotubes could serve as nano-fluidic filtration elements in such applications.

Bionanotechnology could also be very useful in the treatment of the process of membrane biofouling in which microorganisms such as bacteria, fungi, and mold accumulate on the membrane surface. The use of biological materials which are embedded in the filter and do not allow the growth of a microbial population is highly desirable. The anti-biofouling effect could be achieved by the nano-scale organization of physical or (bio)chemical agents which inhibit the growth of the bacteria. Alternatively, slow release from nano-capsules may be used for the treatment.

Another important aspect in the application of biotechnology and nano-technology in water technology is the monitoring of water quality. It is important to monitor both the level of biological and chemical agents, which could be added to the water in a malicious act. They could also be the by-product of the desalination process such as in the case of high levels of boron or radioactive salts when water from a well, rather than seawater, is the initial source for the desalinated water.

8.8. Nanocosmetics

Another interesting application of nanotechnology which may represent a huge market is nanocosmetics. One of the desired applications by the cosmetics companies is to be able to supply the human skin with elements which are associated with a younger appearance and physiological properties. This includes the introduction of various nourishing elements such as vitamins (e.g., the antioxidant lipophilic vitamin E which is limited to oral delivery), cofactors (such as Q10), and even proteins (such as collagen fibrils).

The use of nano-carriers appears a very attractive means of applying such agents to the human skin. The cosmetics industry already utilizes liposomes as carriers of biomolecules to the skin. The use of liposome was reported back in 1986 as part of the Capture® cosmetic formulation of Dior. Just as has been described for the drug delivery applications in the previous chapter, the liposomes serve as containers which allow the delivery of a cargo to the desired part that is being topically treated.

Yet, the use of liposomes is limited only to hydrophilic water-soluble substances as hydrophobic materials can affect the integrity of the liposomes whose self-assembly is driven by hydrophobic interactions. For these applications peptide-based materials, especially those that use electrostatic interactions as the driving force for assembly, may actually be much more attractive vehicles for such topical dermal delivery.

8.9. Solar Energy Applications

The use of bionanotechnology is also envisioned in the field of solar energy. The utilization of solar energy is always a very attractive field of research as the global energy consumption could be accommodated by solar energy if efficient devices were available. Unlike fossil fuel-based energy or atomic energy, solar energy is clean, inexpensive, and environmentally friendly. The recent increase in the price of oil and the declining amount of global reserves make the quest for alternative forms of energy (including geothermal and wind-based energy) very active.

The current photovoltaic solar cells are based on solid-state devices which allow the conversion of photons into a flow of electrons between doped semiconductor cells. One of the limiting factors in the utilization of solar energy is the efficiency of the commercial photocells which is about 10 %. Due to the crucial importance of solar energy, substantial effort is being invested in nanotechnology in general to improve the efficiency of such devices in converting the sun photon flow into an electric current. This includes new types of organic semiconductors and the use of titanium oxide nano-porous materials or quantum dots instead of semiconductor crystals. This is a very intriguing prospect which allows the improvement of research devices to over 30 %. Since the breakthrough of "dye-sensitized solar cells" invented by Michael Graetzel, light harvesting dyes are used in combination with titanium dioxide nanoparticles (Gratzel, 2009).

Biology may actually offer a much better improvement of solar energy efficiency. As all readers know, one of the essences of life is the conversion of solar energy into chemical energy via the process of photosynthesis. This process occurs in plants as well as in photosynthetic bacteria. The process was optimized through billions of years of evolution and the photosystem is the nanobiological assembly which facilitates the harvesting of light and its conversation into chemical energy. The system has the incredible quantum efficiency of 1.0, which means that every photon harvested by the system is converted into an excited state electron. There have been several bionanotechnological attempts to integrate photosynthetic systems into solar cells. The use of proteins from photosynthetic bacteria which could withstand extreme conditions is highly desirable.

Figure 8.3:   Biomolecular solar cell. As in silicon and other semiconductor-based photovoltaic cells, the biomolecular solar cell is based on the flow of electrons by the excitation of a semiconductive material by electromagnetic radiation. The biological photosystem can significantly improve the efficiency of photon collection from solar radiation.

The group of Shuguang Zhang from MIT, mentioned earlier for his seminal work on the self-assembly of peptides, has already demonstrated the proof of this principle by using biological photosystem assemblies in solar cells (Das *et al.*, 2004; Kiley *et al.*, 2005). The researchers created a dense layer of light harvesting system molecules on another layer of organic semiconductor film which was itself on a metal electrode.

Other directions concentrate on the use of small light harvesting molecules called porphyrins which exist in natural photosystems. Of particular interest is the use of self-assembled supramolecular assemblies as templates for the nano-scale organization of porphyrins, in order to facilitate long-range energy transfer. Viruses or self-assembling peptides can be used as such templates (Nam *et al.*, 2010). The diphenylalanine peptides have recently been used as scaffolds for porphyrins, either in a non-covalent co-assembly approach (Kim *et al.*, 2012), or as covalently synthesized F-F-porphyrin building blocks (Charalambidis *et al.*, 2011), with encouraging results.

Chapter 9

Future Prospects for Nanobiotechnology and Bionanotechnology

Nanobiotechnology and bionanotechnology are new scientific disciplines which are still in their infancy. While the prospects discussed throughout this book are enormous and unimaginable, many more directions are yet to be explored. In this chapter we will briefly discuss some of the directions envisioned for the years to come. Some of the directions are straightforward but others are visionary. We will begin with simple directions such as the marriage of genetic engineering and nanotechnology and the extension of the chemical horizons, while we will be concluding with some directions that may still be considered as "science fiction" rather than pure science.

9.1. The Marriage of Molecular Biology and Nanotechnology

There is no dispute that molecular biology had a central role during the second half of the 20th century. While the previous century started with a true revolution in physics, its second half was dominated by the biological revolution. The ability to easily determine the DNA sequence of many organisms, the ability to clone DNA sequences followed by the expression and manipulation of protein and RNA molecules are just a few examples. The budget of biological research in the USA and the rest of the world is continuously growing while the funding of other subjects slowly decreases. The ratio between the funding of NIH (National Institutes of Health) to NASA (National Aeronautics and Space Administration) is one of the indicators of this trend. In the 1960s, the funding for both agencies was about the same; as of 2012 the budget of NIH is almost twice that of NASA (about 32 billion dollars for NIH and 18.7 billion dollars for

NASA). Furthermore, many of the physical science and engineering departments, even including mechanical engineering or electrical engineering departments in traditionally engineering institutes such as the Massachusetts Institute of Technology (MIT) and California Institute of Technology (CalTech), include biological research. Academic departments in areas such as chemistry or materials science are of course even further associated with biological research. Therefore, as has happened in many other areas, the academic world is already integrating the physical and biological sciences. The same union can also be observed in the commercial world. As seen in Appendix B, many companies, large and small, conduct commercial endeavors reflecting the convergence of these two activities. Large semiconductor companies, such as Motorola, initiated activities with very dominant biological relevance.

9.2. The Engineering of Modified Biological Systems for the Assembly of Nano-Structures

As discussed earlier in this book, the field of bionanotechnology is mainly based on the use of natural molecules, mostly DNA or proteins, and small peptide fragments. One area which has not been fully explored is the combination of molecular biology and genetic engineering techniques together with the study of self-assembled biological building blocks. Molecular biology and genetic engineering may allow the integration of various biological functions into self-assembled protein structures. The formation of structures in which biological functions are integrated into nano-structures may be a central theme in the future. In principle it could allow the fabrication not only of well-structured assemblies at the nano-scale, but the formation of such structures which have functional units arranged at a nano-scale order. Enzymes and fluorescent proteins can be genetically fused to self-assembling sequences with the fusion proteins aggregating into inclusion bodies or insoluble fibrils. However, it was proven that in many cases the fibrils form a central "spine" with the enzyme moieties protruding and retaining their activity (Baxa *et al.*, 2003; Mitraki, 2010). This could result in the ability to fabricate structures such as nano-assembly lines in which various changes in a specific molecule could be carried out at nano-scale dimensions. We envision a situation in which the bionanotechnological engineer will be able to design a logical scheme for a systematic and reproducible fabrication of biological-based nanotechnological devices.

The field of nanobiotechnology on the other hand should also be significantly advanced by the marriage between concepts and tools from the physical sciences and molecular biology. Various techniques which were developed and are being developed for non-biological applications could be extremely useful for biological research. Many of the applications which are routinely used in molecular biology could become much more efficient and robust through the use of nanotechnology. DNA manipulation and amplification, a very labor-intensive practice could be dramatically revolutionized by the use of microfluidics and "lab-on-a-chip" techniques. We can envision a situation in which the manipulation of a DNA sample could be automatically performed on a chip in a sequential series of manipulations of a nano-fabricated chip. Another big challenge in the years to come will be the convergence of "top-down" and "bottom-up" approaches towards new generations of devices. Proof-of-principle was recently made for self-assembling peptides and proteins combined with traditional top-down techniques such as microcontact printing, inkjet printing, chemical vapor deposition, and microfluidics (Castillo *et al.*, 2009; Lakshmanan *et al.*, 2012; Shklovsky *et al.*, 2010; Smith *et al.*, 2011).

9.3. Nanotechnology and Tissue Engineering

Tissue engineering is one of the most fascinating directions of modern biotechnology. The term "tissue engineering" was coined by Robert S. Langer from MIT (Langer, 2000) and refers to the ability to engineer and manufacture complete human tissues *in vitro*. The principle of the field of tissue engineering is based on the ability to grow a network of cells, from patients themselves or donors, which will form functional tissues. This tissue could be used later for transplantation in human patients. The ability to conduct such manipulation should drastically change many medical practices and make some of the most severe disorders part of the past. The ability, for example, to make an artificial pancreas in the laboratory will make type I diabetes (juvenile diabetes) a completely curable disorder. Moreover, it may transform pancreatic cancer, one of the most devastating forms of cancer

Figure 9.1: The use of a molecular scaffold for the growth of cells in a three-dimensional matrix could serve as the basis for tissue engineering applications. The control of the tissue morphology and functioning by directing elements and modulating factors is highly desirable.

with extremely poor prognosis of only a few months of survival, into a curable state. Other major tissues which might be engineered include the liver, heart, and kidney. All of these organs are currently only repaired in the human body by transplantation. Yet, there is a chronic lack of organs for transplantation and this process bears many complications due to the immune process. As stated above, one of the major abilities of bionanotechnology is to use the patient's own cells as the mother cells for the engineered tissues. The resulting artificial tissue should therefore have the same immunological parameters as a "self" tissue and rejection should not be an issue anymore.

The basic premise of nanotechnology is to be able to fabricate a "smart matrix" with nano-scale order and signals for the proliferation and differentiation of the cells (Figure 9.1). This matrix will serve as a scaffold for the positioning of stem cells (either embryonic or adult stem cells) and providing them with the right conditions for the development of the engineered organs. The stem cells are unique in their ability to differentiate into cells with very different functional abilities. As all the genetic information exists in each and every cell, stem cells have the potential and the molecular information to become very distinct in their function, synthetic abilities, sensory abilities, and morphology. Some studies suggest the ability to control cell differentiation by external electrical signals will achieve a way in which the process of organ formation is well controlled. Micro- and nano-fabrication techniques can produce biomaterials with controlled topography and mechanical properties; in combination with controlled synthetic micro-environments, these materials can control stem cell differentiation in clinically relevant ways (Fisher *et al.*, 2010).

The use of polymeric scaffolds for the manipulation of tissue has already been demonstrated in the case of cartilage. In most elderly individuals the cartilage tissue is damaged. The dietary supplement of glucosamine and chondroitin sulfate may provide an improvement of the situation, but is far from being a complete solution. The cartilage tissue on the other hand is quite simple and no complex differentiation steps take place. Therefore, the engineering of cartilage tissue was one of the first targets to tackle. Cartilage cells were taken from a patient, grown in tissue culture conditions and then re-transplanted to the same individual. This prevented all forms of immunological rejection and allowed rapid functioning of the transplanted tissue. One of the major tasks of modern nanotechnology is to undertake such practices in more complex organs, such as the heart or liver, in which the spatial organization of the cells and their differentiation according to a planned scheme is much more important.

In some other cases, the ability of tissue regeneration may be a hidden function in the human body and nano-ordered materials could help to execute these abilities. This is especially true for injuries to the nervous system. It is argued that physical support, correct spatial engineering of cell proliferation signals, and biodegradability of engineered biomaterial could allow recovery after spinal cord or optical nerve injuries if applied soon after the injury. If this can be achieved it could pave the way for the transplantation of sensory organs, most importantly the eye. The source of the eyes could come from donors or even tissue-engineered when the technology will allow. Materials that afford nano-scale control such as carbon nanotubes, self-assembling peptides and amphiphiles are increasingly used as scaffolds for cell proliferation and tissue engineering with promising applications (Matson and Stupp, 2012; Wu *et al.*, 2012). These include *in vivo* optical nerve repair (Ellis-Behnke *et al.*, 2006) and central nervous system (CNS) regeneration after chronic injury (Liang *et al.*, 2011).

9.4. Engineering of the Brain Tissue

Another major tissue engineering direction which is discussed less often, but is of enormous medical importance, is the formation of brain tissue in the test tube. The formation of such structures is of course very fascinating as it can provide a cure for devastating diseases such as Alzheimer's disease and Parkinson's disease. As discussed in Chapter 3, these diseases are associated with the self-assembly of amyloid fibrils resulting in the death of the surrounding tissue. These diseases represent a major medical problem; it is estimated that as of 2012 there are about 5.4 million Americans affected by Alzheimer's disease. A similar situation exists in the rest of the world. Since they are associated with advanced age, it is assumed that as life expectancy increases, so will amyloid-related diseases.

We currently understand quite well how to grow individual nerve cells in a tissue culture, but the big challenge is to make it into a functional tissue. Here again, as discussed in the previous section, one of the directions under investigation is the organization of brain cells into a smart polymeric matrix, in which intercellular axonal connections will be directed by the spatial organization of signals. Recently, materials with nano-scale topography which also combine the possibility for electrical or chemical stimulation are being investigated as potential scaffolds for neural regeneration. For example, zinc oxide nanofibers embedded in a polymeric matrix can be implanted and produce an electrical stimulus elicited by ultrasound deformation (Seil and Webster, 2010).

Another approach for the engineering of neural cells is a truly nano-biotechnological one (Fromherz 2002, Kaul *et al.*, 2004). In this approach, nerve cells are deposited on silicon substrates which are litho-graphically defined and the electrical activity of the cells is studied. The basic premise is to be able to form networks that will be complex enough to execute computational tasks. The "brain-chip interfaces" (BCHI) are defined as "hybrid systems where brain cells and chip-based micro-electro-mechanical systems (MEMSs) establish a close physical interaction allowing the transfer of information in one or both directions". BCHIs are increasingly used as implantable microchips for recording or stimulating neuronal excitation and are being investigated for therapeutic purposes (Vassanelli *et al.*, 2012). The final goal is to be able to create some kind of a biological computer out of a silicon chip. This of course has great potential but also many very dangerous aspects as will be briefly discussed in the next chapter.

9.5. Making Artificial Biological Inorganic Composites

As the formation of functioning tissues represents true biological importance, it is no less important to be able to create functional bioinorganic composites. These include artificial bones and teeth. As was discussed earlier, biomineralization represents a major activity in biological systems as well as in artificial nanobiotechnological applications. Therefore the directions which were explored and exploited by the *in vitro* systems may be further developed for the bioengineering of such tissues. Other directions may be different from the replication or mimicking of the calcium-based biomineralization. This could include nano-systems which are based on metals such as platinum and titanium that are currently used for the engineering of macroscopic transplanted objects.

Nanotechnology offers the ability to combine well-ordered structures at the nano-scale, the ordering of inorganic materials such as calcium and its derivatives, the ability to introduce biological signals, and materials of exceptional mechanical rigidity and chemical stability. For example, implant materials can be surface functionalized with either cell adhesive or antifouling motifs using inorganic binding peptides as linkers, resulting in multi-material implants targeted for applications (Khatayevich *et al.*, 2010).

9.6. Nanobio Machines and Nano-Robots

The ultimate goal of nanobiotechnology is the production of functional biologically relevant machines at the nano-scale. Such machines should be able to replace microsurgery by using the submicrometer precision of surgical procedures. One can envision the engineering of tiny robots that will have the cellular dimensions of microns and actual surgical scalpels with submicromic dimensions. Such micro/nanosurgery robots could revolutionize the field of neurosurgery by allowing a very accurate manipulation of the damaged tissue, as in brain tumors or damaged blood vessels, without affecting the healthy tissue. Complicated brain surgery procedures which often end in serious and irreversible complications may be performed by such nano-robots. The idea of nano-robots was indeed the subject of science fiction as in the 1966 classic *Fantastic Voyage* by Isaac Asimov, in which what we would call now a "nano-robot" was introduced into the body of one of the characters and used to destroy a life-threatening blood clot in the brain.

Nano-robots could also be used for the treatment of disorders such as cancer on the cellular level. The key events in the transformation of normal cells into cancerous ones are the mutations within the DNA sequence of affected individuals. For example, most human cancers are associated with a mutation in the gene that encodes the p53 tumor suppressor proteins. Correction of the function of this tumor suppressor, by protein fragments or small molecules, is indeed considered for future therapies. However, other directions are possible; one such direction that still sounds like science fiction is using nano-machines to detect the mutated DNA sequence, binding into the altered sequence, and then correcting the DNA sequence in mutated cancerous cells by nano-scale resolution chemical correction.

Chapter 10

Concluding Remarks: The Prospects and Dangers of the Nanobiological Revolution

There is no task more intellectually challenging than to forecast the future. No one back in the 1950s could even imagine the technological and cultural revolution that would be created by the introduction of personal computers and the Internet. The iPhone was released only in 2007 and nowadays it seems to be an integral part of the technological arena. Nevertheless, without being able to grasp the full scale of future events, it was already very clear by 1950 that the second half of the 20th century would be dominated by electronics and global telecommunication. When we now forecast the second decade of the 21st century and attempt to have some insight into the future it is very clear that the next 50 years will be dominated by a rapid and revolutionary advancement in both the fields of biology and nanotechnology. The fine details are yet to be revealed but the general framework can already be seen. Biology in the first decade of the 21st century is positioned approximately at the same place physics was situated several decades or even a century ago. The general concepts are known, due to an explosion in the amount of experimental information, and there is even significant theoretical understanding of the processes. Most importantly, there is an immense interest and excitement regarding the importance of these studies among the general public as well as among the world leaders and decision-makers.

One fascinating example was the press conference held simultaneously across the Atlantic by Bill Clinton and Tony Blair at the end the 1990s. During this conference they announced the successful completion of the human genome DNA sequencing project and discussed the implications of the project on the future of the citizens of the world. As of

2012, it is almost within reach for each individual to have the full sequence of his or her genome at a cost that is only a tiny fraction of the costs back in the 1990s. In spite of all the excitement and achievements, the pieces of this complicated jigsaw puzzle are not all in their right place and much more needs to be learned in the next 50 years. If we borrow the terminology that was used for physics a century ago, the world of biology is ready for the transition from classical biology into modern biology. Theories that are equivalent in their effect and magnitude to the theories of relativity and quantum mechanics are about to be discovered and formulated. The paradigm of physics research is a very good model for the comprehension of the process of the advancement of science in general and biology in particular. Physics underwent the progression from a discipline dominated by the accumulation of empirical data, and fitting it to simple mathematical models, into a scientific field that allows deep theoretical understanding of very complex processes with an incredibly strong prediction power. Many of the universal parameters, which were predicted theoretically by Einstein's theory of relativity, proved to be accurate only years later. Biology, as the central scientific discipline of the 21st century, is about to undergo the same conceptual revolution. The combination of biology together with nanotechnology should allow the application of physical and technological principles to the study of complex living systems. As discussed throughout this book, biology represents by far the most advanced collection of nano-devices, nano-assemblies and nano-machines.

When we discuss biology as a scientific field, it can be viewed from several different angles and levels. The very basic level is the discovery and formulation of the rules which govern the function of every living cell in both physiological and pathological states. There is a need to understand at the deepest level what makes cells live, divide, function, and die. What is the complete cascade of events which dictate the progression and fate of a living cell? What makes one cell different from the other? What makes the same cell function differently in one person compared with another? What is going wrong when a normal cell is transformed into a malignant cell? Why is a newly divided cell different in an older person compared with a young person or a newborn? This is only a very partial list of the different questions that fascinates every researcher and every person who is concerned about the meaning of life. As mentioned above, many of the details are known, but the outcome of the emerging fields of genomics and proteomics will provide the field with a much deeper and more complete understanding. The completion of the human genome project is certainly a pivotal milestone in that direction. The next step will be the sequencing of the genomes of every individual and of any known species on Earth. Such information will allow us to realize the similarities and differences between living individuals and will put the field of genetics in a completely new light. Nevertheless, the mere knowledge of the DNA sequences is not enough. A common analogy often made is that just looking at the list of parts of a Boeing 747 jet does not give a person who has never seen a plane even the faintest hint about the way that this mammoth can fly. The next step in our understanding of the secrets of life is to study the main products of the genes: the proteins. This emerging field is called proteomics. The study of proteomics brings us one level higher. However, even this is not enough and we should obtain information about the map of the interaction between proteins, their structure and folding, and their ability to specifically interact with the DNA, which controls the flow of information from the genome to the cells.

The next step after the understanding of the building blocks on the one hand and the method of assembly and function on the other will be the engineering of such activities. The prospects for the combination of the fabrication abilities and patterning as we learn from nanotechnology together with the understanding of the biological function can be revolutionary. Will we be able to design and manufacture living organisms as we design computers today? Can we manipulate living organisms as easily as we design integrated electronic circuits? These questions and others will be answered in years to come.

One of the most intriguing enigmas in biology is the function of the brain. In its essence, the study of the brain aims towards the understanding of the biochemical and molecular basis of thinking and reasoning. The brain is certainly the masterpiece of biological creation and the biggest mystery of all. Computers can calculate much faster than humans, and they can remember billions of phone numbers and financial transactions. However, no computer can think and no computer can make a moral decision. Above all, no computer can really perform a true recognition process that any young child can. Any four-year-old child can easily distinguish between a horse and a donkey. This simple task cannot be truly performed by a supercomputer with the most sophisticated software and hardware. There has been significant advancement in the field of artificial intelligence using new mathematical tools such as fuzzy logic and neural networks. These methods were developed with the aim of mimicking the computational process of the brain. However, with all the advancements in those fields, the most modern supercomputer cannot even compete with a young toddler or even a fruit fly. The reason for this is probably due to the fact that all these methods are missing some of the very fundamental concepts of brain function. In our opinion, in the particular field of brain and cognition studies, we are still waiting for a completely new and revolutionary theory, in the same conceptual magnitude as the theories of relativity or quantum mechanics. Only such a revolutionary theory will be able to truly explain the process of thinking. On the way to the breakthrough theory, nano-science and nanotechnology can play a central role. We would like to know about the molecular details of being mentally retarded or a genius. What is the net difference in the brain of a mouse before and after it knows the way through the maze in order to get to the piece of cheese? Moreover, will we be able to use technology, most interestingly nanotechnology, to fabricate an artificial brain, a genuine artificial intelligence device?

Many people ask themselves whether machines will ever have the ability to think. The answer is very clear and simple: there are machines that can think! The most elaborate example is called *Homo sapiens*. Unless we fully accept Descartes's body and mind dualism, there is no choice but to state that the brain is a machine that can think and that this thinking is performed by the use of basic and finite chemical processes. The brain is a very elaborate machine, but it is just a machine which obeys the rules of chemistry and physics. There is no reason that such a machine will not eventually be built in a laboratory or even in a mass production assembly line. The bionanotechnological principles presented in this book allow us to envision ways to make such complex machines by understanding the principles and practice of the assembly of a complex network of biological neurons into a silico-biological artificial device.

Finally, a few last words about the dangers of bionanotechnology and nanobiotechnology. Here, at the end of the book, we come back to the parallels between biology and physics. The most dangerous outcome of modern physics was the atomic bomb. There has always been a great fear of a Third World War in which atomic weapons will be used to destroy the world. Only a very fine network of checks and balances as well as the general understanding of the horrible outcome of the use of the bomb saves us from devastation. The harmful potential of the nanotechnological revolution is no smaller than that posed by atomic weapons. In fact, it is much more dangerous. It is our duty to make sure that the nanotechnological tools will be used only for the best.

Appendix A

There's Plenty of Room at the Bottom: An Invitation to Enter a New Field of Physics — by Richard P. Feynman

The transcript of the original talk by Richard Feynman is reproduced with permission from the *Engineering & Science* magazine, California Institute of Technology, Volume 23, Number 5, February 1960. It is presented to the readers as a vivid illustration of the imagination and vision of one of the greatest scientific leaders of the 20th century.

Although the term "nanotechnology" is not mentioned in this lecture (as discussed in Chapter 2, it was suggested several years later), the address is certainly the cornerstone of modern nanotechnology. It is quite astonishing how well Feynman's remarks are still relevant almost half a century after his original address. As discussed previously, one of the most interesting things related to the readers of this book is Feynman's vision regarding the field of biology. Unlike many physicists of his time, Feynman understood how important biology is in the framework of nanotechnology.

There's Plenty of Room at the Bottom: An Invitation to Enter a New Field of Physics

Richard P. Feynman

I imagine experimental physicists must often look with envy at men like Kamerlingh Onnes, who discovered a field like low temperature, which seems to be bottomless and in which one can go down and down.

Such a man is then a leader and has some temporary monopoly in a scientific adventure. Percy Bridgman, in designing a way to obtain higher pressures, opened up another new field and was able to move into it and to lead us all along. The development of an ever higher vacuum was a continuing development of the same kind.

I would like to describe a field, in which little has been done, but in which an enormous amount can be done in principle. This field is not quite the same as the others in that it will not tell us much of fundamental physics (in the sense of, "What are the strange particles?"), but it is more like solid-state physics in the sense that it might tell us much of great interest about the strange phenomena that occur in complex situations. Furthermore, a point that is most important is that it would have an enormous number of technical applications.

What I want to talk about is the problem of manipulating and controlling things on a small scale.

As soon as I mention this, people tell me about miniaturization, and how far it has progressed today. They tell me about electric motors that are the size of the nail on your small finger. And there is a device on the market, they tell me, by which you can write the Lord's Prayer on the head of a pin. But that's nothing; that's the most primitive, halting step in the direction I intend to discuss. It is a staggeringly small world that is below. In the year 2000, when they look back at this age, they will wonder why it was not until the year 1960 that anybody began seriously to move in this direction.

Why cannot we write the entire 24 volumes of the Encyclopaedia Britannica on the head of a pin?

Let's see what would be involved. The head of a pin is a sixteenth of an inch across. If you magnify it by 25,000 diameters, the area of the head of the pin is then equal to the area of all the pages of the Encyclopaedia Britannica. Therefore, all it is necessary to do is to reduce in size all the writing in the Encyclopaedia by 25,000 times. Is that possible? The resolving power of the eye is about 1/120 of an inch — that is roughly the diameter of one of the little dots on the fine half-tone reproductions in the Encyclopaedia. This, when you demagnify it by 25,000 times, is still 80 angstroms in diameter — 32 atoms across, in an ordinary metal. In other words, one of those dots still would contain in its area 1,000 atoms. So, each dot can easily be adjusted in size as required by the photoengraving, and there is no question that there is enough room on the head of a pin to put all of the Encyclopaedia Britannica.

Furthermore, it can be read if it is so written. Let's imagine that it is written in raised letters of metal; that is, where the black is in the Encyclopaedia, we have raised letters of metal that are actually 1/25,000 of their ordinary size. How would we read it?

If we had something written in such a way, we could read it using techniques in common use today. (They will undoubtedly find a better way when we do actually have it written, but to make my point conservatively I shall just take techniques we know today.) We would press the metal into a plastic material and make a mold of it, then peel the plastic off very carefully, evaporate silica into the plastic to get a very thin film, then shadow it by evaporating gold at an angle against the silica so that all the little letters will appear clearly, dissolve the plastic away from the silica film, and then look through it with an electron microscope!

There is no question that if the thing were reduced by 25,000 times in the form of raised letters on the pin, it would be easy for us to read it today. Furthermore, there is no question that we would find it easy to make copies of the master; we would just need to press the same metal plate again into plastic and we would have another copy.

How do we write small?

The next question is: how do we *write* it? We have no standard technique to do this now. But let me argue that it is not as difficult as it first appears to be. We can reverse the lenses of the electron microscope in order to demagnify as well as magnify. A source of ions, sent through the microscope lenses in reverse, could be focused to a very small spot. We could write with that spot like we write in a TV cathode ray oscilloscope, by going across in lines, and having an adjustment which determines the amount of material which is going to be deposited as we scan in lines.

This method might be very slow because of space charge limitations. There will be more rapid methods. We could first make, perhaps by some photo process, a screen which has holes in it in the form of the letters. Then we would strike an arc behind the holes and draw metallic ions through the holes; then we could again use our system of lenses and make a small image in the form of ions, which would deposit the metal on the pin.

A simpler way might be this (though I am not sure it would work): we take light and, through an optical microscope running backwards, we focus it onto a very small photoelectric screen. Then electrons come away from the screen where the light is shining. These electrons are focused down in size by the electron microscope lenses to impinge directly upon the surface of the metal. Will such a beam etch away the metal if it is run long enough? I don't know. If it doesn't work for a metal surface, it must be possible to find some surface with which to coat the original pin so that, where the electrons bombard, a change is made which we could recognize later.

There is no intensity problem in these devices — not what you are used to in magnification, where you have to take a few electrons and spread them over a bigger and bigger screen; it is just the opposite. The light which we get from a page is concentrated onto a very small area so it is very intense. The few electrons which come from the photoelectric screen are demagnified down to a very tiny area so that, again, they are very intense. I don't know why this hasn't been done yet!

That's the Encyclopaedia Britannica on the head of a pin, but let's consider all the books in the world. The Library of Congress has approximately 9 million volumes; the British Museum Library has five million volumes; there are also 5 million volumes in the National Library in France. Undoubtedly there are duplications, so let us say that there are some 24 million volumes of interest in the world.

What would happen if I print all this down at the scale we have been discussing? How much space would it take? It would take, of course, the area of about a million pinheads because, instead of there being just the 24 volumes of the Encyclopaedia, there are 24 million volumes. The million pinheads can be put in a square of a thousand pins on a side, or an area of about 3 square yards. That is to say, the silica replica with the paper-thin backing of plastic, with which we have made the copies, with all this information, is on an area of approximately the size of 35 pages of the Encyclopaedia. That is about half as many pages as there are in this magazine. All of the information which all of mankind has ever recorded in books can be carried around in a pamphlet in your hand — and not written in code, but a simple reproduction of the original pictures, engravings, and everything else on a small scale without loss of resolution.

What would our librarian at Caltech say, as she runs all over from one building to another, if I tell her that, ten years from now, all of the information that she is struggling to keep track of — 120,000 volumes, stacked from the floor to the ceiling, drawers full of cards, storage rooms full of the older books — can be kept on just one library card! When the University of Brazil, for example, finds that their library is burned, we can send them a copy of every book in our library by striking off a copy from the master plate in a few hours and mailing it in an envelope no bigger or heavier than any other ordinary airmail letter.

Now, the name of this talk is "There is *Plenty* of Room at the Bottom" — not just "There is Room at the Bottom." What I have demonstrated is that there *is* room — that you can decrease the size of things in a practical way. I now want to show that there is *plenty* of room. I will not now discuss how we are going to do it, but only what is possible in principle — in other words, what is possible according to the laws of physics. I am not inventing antigravity, which is possible someday only if the laws are not what we think. I am telling you what could be done if the laws *are* what we think; we are not doing it simply because we haven't yet gotten around to it.

Information on a small scale

Suppose that, instead of trying to reproduce the pictures and all the information directly in its present form, we write only the information content in a code of dots and dashes, or something like that, to represent the various letters. Each letter represents six or seven "bits" of information; that is, you need only about six or seven dots or dashes for each letter. Now, instead of writing everything, as I did before, on the *surface* of the head of a pin, I am going to use the interior of the material as well.

Let us represent a dot by a small spot of one metal, the next dash, by an adjacent spot of another metal, and so on. Suppose, to be conservative, that a bit of information is going to require a little cube of atoms $5 \times 5 \times 5$ that is 125 atoms. Perhaps we need a hundred and some odd atoms to make sure that the information is not lost through diffusion, or through some other process.

I have estimated how many letters there are in the Encyclopaedia, and I have assumed that each of my 24 million books is as big as an Encyclopaedia volume, and have calculated, then, how many bits of information there are (10^{15}). For each bit I allow 100 atoms. And it turns out that all of the information that man has carefully accumulated in all the books in the world can be written in this form in a cube of material one two-hundredth of an inch wide — which is the barest piece of dust that can be made out by the human eye. So there is *plenty* of room at the bottom! Don't tell me about microfilm!

This fact — that enormous amounts of information can be carried in an exceedingly small space — is, of course, well known to the biologists, and resolves the mystery which existed before we understood all this clearly, of how it could be that, in the tiniest cell, all of the information for the organization of a complex creature such as ourselves can be stored. All this information — whether we have brown eyes, or whether we think at all, or that in the embryo the jawbone should first develop with a little hole in the side so that later a nerve can grow through it — all this information is contained in a very tiny fraction of the cell in the form of long-chain DNA molecules in which approximately 50 atoms are used for one bit of information about the cell.

Better electron microscopes

If I have written in a code, with $5 \times 5 \times 5$ atoms to a bit, the question is: how could I read it today? The electron microscope is not quite good enough, with the greatest care and effort it can only resolve about 10 angstroms. I would like to try and impress upon you while I am talking about all of these things on a small scale, the importance of improving the electron microscope by a hundred times. It is not impossible; it is not against the laws of diffraction of the electron. The wavelength of the electron in such a microscope is only 1/20 of an angstrom. So it should be possible to see the individual atoms. What good would it be to see individual atoms distinctly?

We have friends in other fields — in biology, for instance. We physicists often look at them and say, "You know the reason you fellows are making so little progress?" (Actually I don't know any field where they are making more rapid progress than they are in biology today.) "You should use more mathematics, like we do." They could answer us — but they're polite, so I'll answer for them: "What *you* should do in order for *us* to make more rapid progress is to make the electron microscope 100 times better."

What are the most central and fundamental problems of biology today? They are questions like: what is the sequence of bases in the DNA? What happens when you have a mutation? How is the base order in the DNA connected to the order of amino acids in the protein? What is the structure of the RNA; is it single chain or double chain, and how is it related in its order of bases to the DNA? What is the organization of the microsomes? How are proteins synthesized? Where does the RNA go? How does it sit? Where do the proteins sit? Where do the amino acids go in? In photosynthesis, where is the chlorophyll; how is it arranged; where are the carotenoids involved in this thing? What is the system of the conversion of light into chemical energy?

It is very easy to answer many of these fundamental biological questions; *you just look at the thing!* You will see the order of bases in the chain; you will see the structure of the microsome. Unfortunately, the present microscope sees at a scale which is just a bit too crude. Make the microscope 100 times more powerful, and many problems of biology would be made very much easier. I exaggerate, of course, but the biologists would surely be very thankful to you — and they would prefer that to the criticism that they should use more mathematics.

The theory of chemical processes today is based on theoretical physics. In this sense, physics supplies the foundation of chemistry. But chemistry also has analysis. If you have a strange substance and you want to know what it is, you go through a long and complicated process of chemical analysis. You can analyze almost anything today, so I am a little late with my idea. But if the physicists wanted to, they could also dig under the chemists in the problem of chemical analysis. It would be very easy to make an analysis of any complicated chemical substance; all one would have to do would be to look at it and see where the atoms are. The only trouble is that the electron microscope is 100 times too poor. (Later, I would like to ask the question: can the physicists do something about the third problem of chemistry — namely, synthesis? Is there a *physical* way to synthesize any chemical substance?)

The reason the electron microscope is so poor is that the f-value of the lenses is only 1 part to 1,000; you don't have a big enough numerical aperture. And I know that there are theorems which prove that it is impossible, with axially symmetrical stationary field lenses, to produce an f-value any bigger than so and so; and therefore the resolving power at the present time is at its theoretical maximum. But in every theorem there are assumptions. Why must the field be symmetrical? I put this out as a challenge: is there no way to make the electron microscope more powerful?

The marvelous biological system

The biological example of writing information on a small scale has inspired me to think of something that should be possible. Biology is not simply writing information; it is *doing something* about it. A biological system can be exceedingly small. Many of the cells are very tiny, but they are very active; they manufacture various substances; they walk around; they wiggle; and they do all kinds of marvelous things — all on a very small scale. Also, they store information. Consider the possibility that we too can make a thing very small which does what we want — that we can manufacture an object that maneuvers at that level!

There may even be an economic point to this business of making things very small. Let me remind you of some of the problems of computing machines. In computers we have to store an enormous amount of information. The kind of writing that I was mentioning before, in which I had everything down as a distribution of metal, is permanent. Much more interesting to a computer is a way of writing, erasing, and writing something else. (This is usually because we don't want to waste the material on which we have just written. Yet, if we could write it in a very small space, it wouldn't make any difference; it could just be thrown away after it was read. It doesn't cost very much for the material.)

Miniaturizing the computer

I don't know how to do this on a small scale in a practical way, but I do know that computing machines are very large; they fill rooms. Why can't we make them very small, make them of little wires, little elements — and by little, I mean *little*. For instance, the wires should be 10 or 100 atoms in diameter, and the circuits should be a few thousand angstroms across. Everybody who has analyzed the logical theory of computers has come to the conclusion that the possibilities of computers are very interesting — if they could be made to be more complicated by several orders of magnitude. If they had millions of times as many elements, they could make judgments. They would have time to calculate what is the best way to make the calculation that they are about to make. They could select the method of analysis which, from their experience, is better than the one that we would give to them. And in many other ways, they would have new qualitative features.

If I look at your face I immediately recognize that I have seen it before. (Actually, my friends will say I have chosen an unfortunate example here for the subject of this illustration. At least I recognize that it is a *man* and not an *apple*.) Yet, there is no machine which, with that speed, can take a picture of a face and say even that it is a man; and much less that it is the same man that you showed it before — unless it is exactly the same picture. If the face is changed; if I am closer to the face; if I am further from the face; if the light changes — I recognize it anyway. Now, this little computer I carry in my head is easily able to do that. The computers that we build are not able to do that. The number of elements in this bone box of mine are enormously greater than the number of elements in our "wonderful" computers. But our mechanical computers are too big; the elements in this box are microscopic. I want to make some that are submicroscopic.

If we wanted to make a computer that had all these marvelous extra qualitative abilities, we would have to make it, perhaps, the size of the Pentagon. This has several disadvantages. First, it requires too much material; there may not be enough germanium in the world for all the transistors which would have to be put into this enormous thing. There is also the problem of heat generation and power consumption; TVA would be needed to run the computer. But an even more practical difficulty is that the computer would be limited to a certain speed. Because of its large size, there is finite time required to get the information from one place to another. The information cannot go any faster than the speed of light — so, ultimately, when our computers get faster and faster and more and more elaborate, we will have to make them smaller and smaller.

But there is plenty of room to make them smaller. There is nothing that I can see in the physical laws that says the computer elements cannot be made enormously smaller than they are now. In fact, there may be certain advantages.

Miniaturization by evaporation

How can we make such a device? What kind of manufacturing processes would we use? One possibility we might consider, since we have talked about writing by putting atoms down in a certain arrangement, would be to evaporate the material, then evaporate the insulator next to it. Then, for the next layer, evaporate another position of a wire, another insulator, and so on. So, you simply evaporate until you have a block of stuff which has the elements — coils and condensers, transistors and so on — of exceedingly fine dimensions.

But I would like to discuss, just for amusement, that there are other possibilities. Why can't we manufacture these small computers somewhat like we manufacture the big ones? Why can't we drill holes, cut things, solder things, stamp things out, mold different shapes all at an infinitesimal level? What are the limitations as to how small a thing has to be before you can no longer mold it? How many times when you are working on something frustratingly tiny like your wife's wristwatch, have you said to yourself, "If I could only train an ant to do this!" What I would like to suggest is the possibility of training an ant to train a mite to do this. What are the possibilities of small but movable machines? They may or may not be useful, but they surely would be fun to make.

Consider any machine — for example, an automobile — and ask about the problems of making an infinitesimal machine like it. Suppose, in the particular design of the automobile, we need a certain precision of the parts; we need an accuracy, let's suppose, of 4/10,000 of an inch. If things are more inaccurate than that in the shape of the cylinder and so on, it isn't going to work very well. If I make the thing too small, I have to worry about the size of the atoms; I can't make a circle of "balls" so to speak, if the circle is too small. So, if I make the error, corresponding to 4/10,000 of an inch, correspond to an error of ten atoms, it turns out that I can reduce the dimensions of an automobile 4,000 times, approximately — so that it is 1 mm across. Obviously, if you redesign the car so that it would work with a much larger tolerance, which is not at all impossible, then you could make a much smaller device.

It is interesting to consider what the problems are in such small machines. Firstly, with parts stressed to the same degree, the forces go as the area you are reducing, so that things like weight and inertia are of relatively no importance. The strength of material, in other words, is very much greater in proportion. The stresses and expansion of the flywheel from centrifugal force, for example, would be the same proportion only if the rotational speed is increased in the same proportion as we decrease the size. On the other hand, the metals that we use have a grain structure, and this would be very annoying at small scale because the material is not homogeneous. Plastics and glass and things of this amorphous nature are very much more homogeneous, and so we would have to make our machines out of such materials.

There are problems associated with the electrical part of the system — with the copper wires and the magnetic parts. The magnetic properties on a very small scale are not the same as on a large scale; there is the "domain" problem involved. A big magnet made of millions of domains can only be made on a small scale with one domain. The electrical equipment won't simply be scaled down; it has to be redesigned. But I can see no reason why it can't be redesigned to work again.

Problems of lubrication

Lubrication involves some interesting points. The effective viscosity of oil would be higher and higher in proportion as we went down (and if we increase the speed as much as we can). If we don't increase the speed so much, and change from oil to kerosene or some other fluid, the problem is not so bad. But actually we may not have to lubricate at all! We have a lot of extra force. Let the bearings run dry; they won't run hot because the heat escapes away from such a small device very, very rapidly.

This rapid heat loss would prevent the gasoline from exploding, so an internal combustion engine is impossible. Other chemical reactions, liberating energy when cold, can be used. Probably an external supply of electrical power would be most convenient for such small machines.

What would be the utility of such machines? Who knows? Of course, a small automobile would only be useful for the mites to drive around in, and I suppose our Christian interests don't go that far. However, we did note the possibility of the manufacture of small elements for computers in completely automatic factories, containing lathes and other machine tools at the very small level. The small lathe would not have to be exactly like our big lathe. I leave to your imagination the improvement of the design to take full advantage of the properties of things on a small scale, and in such a way that the fully automatic aspect would be easiest to manage.

A friend of mine (Albert R. Hibbs) suggests a very interesting possibility for relatively small machines. He says that, although it is a very wild idea, it would be interesting in surgery if you could swallow the surgeon. You put the mechanical surgeon inside the blood vessel and it goes into the heart and "looks" around. (Of course the information has to be fed out.) It finds out which valve is the faulty one and takes a little knife and slices it out. Other small machines might be permanently incorporated in the body to assist some inadequately functioning organ.

Now comes the interesting question: how do we make such a tiny mechanism? I leave that to you. However, let me suggest one weird possibility. You know, in the atomic energy plants they have materials and machines that they can't handle directly because they have become radioactive. To unscrew nuts and put on bolts and so on, they have a set of master and slave hands, so that by operating a set of levers here, you control the "hands" there, and can turn them this way and that so you can handle things quite nicely.

Most of these devices are actually made rather simply, in that there is a particular cable, like a marionette string, that goes directly from the controls to the "hands". But, of course, things also have been made using servo motors, so that the connection between the one thing and the other is electrical rather than mechanical. When you turn the levers, they turn a servo motor, and it changes the electrical currents in the wires, which repositions a motor at the other end.

Now, I want to build much the same device — a master-slave system which operates electrically. But I want the slaves to be made especially carefully by modern large-scale machinists so that they are one-fourth the scale of the "hands" that you ordinarily maneuver. So you have a scheme by which you can do things at one-quarter scale anyway — the little servo motors with little hands play with little nuts and bolts; they drill little holes; they are four times smaller. Aha! So I manufacture a quarter-size lathe; I manufacture quarter-size tools; and I make, at the one-quarter scale, still another set of hands again relatively one-quarter size! This is one-sixteenth size, from my point of view. And after I finish doing this I wire directly from my large-scale system, through transformers perhaps, to the one-sixteenth size servo motors. Thus I can now manipulate the one-sixteenth size hands.

Well, you get the principle from there on. It is rather a difficult program, but it is a possibility. You might say that one can go much farther in one step than from one to four. Of course, this has all to be designed very carefully and it is not necessary simply to make it like hands. If you thought of it very carefully, you could probably arrive at a much better system for doing such things.

If you work through a pantograph, even today, you can get much more than a factor of four in even one step. But you can't work directly through a pantograph which makes a smaller pantograph which then makes a smaller pantograph — because of the looseness of the holes and the irregularities of construction. The end of the pantograph wiggles with a relatively greater irregularity than the irregularity with which you move your hands. In going down this scale, I would find the end of the pantograph on the end of the pantograph on the end of the pantograph shaking so badly that it wasn't doing anything sensible at all.

At each stage, it is necessary to improve the precision of the apparatus. If, for instance, having made a small lathe with a pantograph, we find its lead screw irregular — more irregular than the large-scale one — we could lap the lead screw against breakable nuts that you can reverse in the usual way back and forth until this lead screw is, at its scale, as accurate as our original lead screws, at our scale.

We can make flats by rubbing unflat surfaces in triplicates together — in three pairs — and the flats then become flatter than the thing you started with. Thus, it is not impossible to improve precision on a small scale by the correct operations. So, when we build this stuff, it is necessary at each step to improve the accuracy of the equipment by working for awhile down there, making accurate lead screws, Johansen blocks, and all the other materials which we use in accurate machine work at the higher level. We have to stop at each level and manufacture all the stuff to go to the next level — a very long and very difficult program. Perhaps you can figure a better way than that to get down to small scale more rapidly.

Yet, after all this, you have just got one little baby lathe four thousand times smaller than usual. But we were thinking of making an enormous computer, which we were going to build by drilling holes on this lathe to make little washers for the computer. How many washers can you manufacture on this one lathe?

A hundred tiny hands

When I make my first set of slave "hands" at one-fourth scale, I am going to make ten sets. I make ten sets of "hands", and I wire them to my original levers so they each do exactly the same thing at the same time in parallel. Now, when I am making my new devices one-quarter again as small, I let each one manufacture ten copies, so that I would have a hundred "hands" at the 1/16th size.

Where am I going to put the million lathes that I am going to have? Why, there is nothing to it; the volume is much less than that of even one full-scale lathe. For instance, if I made a billion little lathes, each 1/4,000 of the scale of a regular lathe, there are plenty of materials and space available because in the billion little ones there is less than 2 percent of the materials in one big lathe.

It doesn't cost anything for materials, you see. So I want to build a billion tiny factories, models of each other, which are manufacturing simultaneously, drilling holes, stamping parts, and so on.

As we go down in size, there are a number of interesting problems that arise. All things do not simply scale down in proportion. There is the problem that materials stick together by the molecular (Van der Waals) attractions. It would be like this: after you have made a part and you unscrew the nut from a bolt, it isn't going to fall down because the gravity isn't appreciable; it would even be hard to get it off the bolt. It would be like those old movies of a man with his hands full of molasses, trying to get rid of a glass of water. There will be several problems of this nature that we will have to be ready to design for.

Rearranging the atoms

But I am not afraid to consider the final question as to whether, ultimately — in the great future — we can arrange the atoms the way we want; the very atoms, all the way down! What would happen if we could arrange the atoms one by one the way we want them (within reason, of course; you can't put them so that they are chemically unstable, for example).

Up to now, we have been content to dig in the ground to find minerals. We heat them and we do things on a large scale with them, and we hope to get a pure substance with just so much impurity, and so on. But we must always accept some atomic arrangement that nature gives us. We haven't got anything, say, with a "checkerboard" arrangement, with the impurity atoms exactly arranged 1,000 angstroms apart, or in some other particular pattern.

What could we do with layered structures with just the right layers? What would the properties of materials be if we could really arrange the atoms the way we want them? They would be very interesting to investigate theoretically. I can't see exactly what would happen, but I can hardly doubt that when we have some control of the arrangement of things on a small scale we will get an enormously greater range of possible properties that substances can have, and of different things that we can do.

Consider, for example, a piece of material in which we make little coils and condensers (or their solid-state analogs) 1,000 or 10,000 angstroms in a circuit, one right next to the other, over a large area, with little antennas sticking out at the other end — a whole series of circuits. Is it possible, for example, to emit light from a whole set of antennas, like we emit radio waves from an organized set of antennas to beam the radio programs to Europe? The same thing would be to beam the light out in a definite direction with very high intensity. (Perhaps such a beam is not very useful technically or economically.)

I have thought about some of the problems of building electric circuits on a small scale, and the problem of resistance is serious. If you build a corresponding circuit on a small scale, its natural frequency goes up, since the wavelength goes down as the scale; but the skin depth only decreases with the square root of the scale ratio, and so resistive problems are of increasing difficulty. Possibly we can beat resistance through the use of superconductivity if the frequency is not too high, or by other tricks.

Atoms in a small world

When we get to the very, very small world — say circuits of seven atoms — we have a lot of new things that would happen that represent completely new opportunities for design. Atoms on a small scale behave like nothing on a large scale, for they satisfy the laws of quantum mechanics. So, as we go down and fiddle around with the atoms down there, we are working with different laws, and we can expect to do different things. We can manufacture in different ways. We can use, not just circuits, but some system involving the quantized energy levels, or the interactions of quantized spins, etc.

Another thing we will notice is that, if we go down far enough, all of our devices can be mass produced so that they are absolutely perfect copies of one another. We cannot build two large machines so that the dimensions are exactly the same. But if your machine is only 100 atoms high, you only have to get it correct to one-half of one percent to make sure the other machine is exactly the same size — namely, 100 atoms high!

At the atomic level, we have new kinds of forces and new kinds of possibilities, new kinds of effects. The problems of manufacture and reproduction of materials will be quite different. I am, as I said, inspired by the biological phenomena in which chemical forces are used in repetitious fashion to produce all kinds of weird effects (one of which is the author).

The principles of physics, as far as I can see, do not speak against the possibility of maneuvering things atom by atom. It is not an attempt to violate any laws; it is something, in principle, that can be done; but in practice, it has not been done because we are too big.

Ultimately, we can do chemical synthesis. A chemist comes to us and says, "Look, I want a molecule that has the atoms arranged thus and so; make me that molecule." The chemist does a mysterious thing when he wants to make a molecule. He sees that it has got that ring, so he mixes this and that, and he shakes it, and he fiddles around. And, at the end of a difficult process, he usually does succeed in synthesizing what he wants. By the time I get my devices working, so that we can do it by physics, he will have figured out how to synthesize absolutely anything, so that this will really be useless.

But it is interesting that it would be, in principle, possible (I think) for a physicist to synthesize any chemical substance that the chemist writes down. Give the orders and the physicist synthesizes it. How? Put the atoms down where the chemist says, and so you make the substance. The problems of chemistry and biology can be greatly helped if our ability to see what we are doing, and to do things on an atomic level, is ultimately developed — a development which I think cannot be avoided.

Now, you might say, "Who should do this and why should they do it?" Well, I pointed out a few of the economic applications, but I know that the reason that you would do it might be just for fun. But have some fun! Let's have a competition between laboratories. Let one laboratory make a tiny motor which it sends to another lab which sends it back with a thing that fits inside the shaft of the first motor.

High school competition

Just for the fun of it, and in order to get kids interested in this field, I would propose that someone who has some contact with the high schools think of making some kind of high school competition. After all, we haven't even started in this field, and even the kids can write smaller than has ever been written before. They could have competition in high schools. The Los Angeles high school could send a pin to the Venice high school on which it says, "How's this?" They get the pin back, and in the dot of the "i" it says, "Not so hot."

Perhaps this doesn't excite you to do it, and only economics will do so. Then I want to do something; but I can't do it at the present moment, because I haven't prepared the ground. It is my intention to offer a prize of $1,000 to the first guy who can take the information on the page of a book and put it on an area 1/25,000 smaller in linear scale in such manner that it can be read by an electron microscope.

And I want to offer another prize — if I can figure out how to phrase it so that I don't get into a mess of arguments about definitions — of another $1,000 to the first guy who makes an operating electric motor — a rotating electric motor which can be controlled from the outside and, not counting the lead-in wires, is only 1/64 inch cube.

I do not expect that such prizes will have to wait very long for claimants.

Appendix B

List of Bionanotechnological
and Nanobiotechnological Companies

The field of nanobiotechnology and bionanotechnology is a very dynamic one. As in other hi-tech commercial activities it combines well-established companies (such as mega-sized chemical manufactures) as well as younger companies and newborn start-ups. Here is a (non-exhaustive) list of active companies as of 2012:

3DM (http://www.puramatrix.com/): The production of self-assembled biomaterials with nano-scale order for the application of tissue engineering and repair.

3DM Inc.
245 First Street
Cambridge, MA 02142, USA
E-mail: contact@puramatrix.com

Ademtech (http://www.ademtech.com/): The production of calibrated magnetic emulsions for *in vitro* diagnosis and life sciences application.

Ademtech
Parc Scientifique Unitec 1
4 Allée du doyen Georges Brus
33600 Pessac, France
E-mail: ademtech@ademtech.com

Alnis BioSciences (http://www.alnis.com/): The production of "engineered nanoscopic hydrogels, or NanoGels, comprised of polymers, bioactives, and targeting molecules. These NanoGels are intended to selectively target pathological tissues, treat the disease, and afterwards simply disintegrate, returning to the individual components from which they were formed".

Alnis BioSciences, Inc.
626 Bancroft Way #3B
Berkeley, CA 94710, USA
E-mail: alnis@alnis.com

Agilent Technologies (spin-off Hewlett-Packard Company) (http://www. agilent.com): Advance measurement tools for life science and medical use.

Agilent Technologies, Inc.
5301 Stevens Creek Blvd
Santa Clara, CA 95051, USA
E-mail: Contact_Us@agilent.com

Artificial Cell Technologies (http://www.artificialcelltech.com/): The production of synthetic vaccines using a technology platform of ultra-thin multilayer polypeptide nanofilms.

Artificial Cell Technologies, Inc.
5 Science Park
New Haven, CT 06511, USA
E-mail: info@artificialcelltech.com

Asklêpios BioPharmaceutical (http://www.askbio.com/): "Biotechnology company engaged in the development and delivery of novel protein and cellular-based therapies through the design of proprietary Biological Nano Particles ('BNP')."

Asklêpios BioPharmaceutical Inc.
45 N. Chatham Parkway
Chapel Hill, NC 27517, USA
E-mail: info@askbio.com

BioCrystal (http://www.biocrystal.com/): Production of nanocrystalline fluorescent markers for cell and intracellular detection and analysis.

BioCrystal, Ltd.
575 McCorkle Boulevard
Westerville, OH 43082, USA
E-mail: info@biocrystal.com

BioForce Nanosciences (http://www.bioforcenano.com/): A nanotechnology company providing innovative nanotech tools and solutions for the life sciences through instruments, consumables, and applications.

BioForce Nanosciences, Inc.
609 E Lincoln Way, Suite 609
Ames, IA 50010, USA
E-mail: info@bioforcenano.com

Dendritech (http://www.dendritech.com/): "Dendritech is a specialty polymer company focused on the development of dendritic, hyperbranched and tailor-made polymer products."

Dendritech, Inc.
3110 Schuette Dr.
Midland, MI 48642, USA
E-mail: scheibert@dendritech.com

Dendritic NanoTechnologies (http://dnanotech.com/): "DNT is the world's leading developer and provider of advanced dendritic polymers, a breakthrough enabling technology that provides the vehicle — the targeting and delivery mechanisms — for a vast array of diagnostic and therapeutics solutions — *in vitro* and *in vivo*."

Dendritic NanoTechnologies Inc.
2625 Denison Dr.
Mount Pleasant, MI 48858, USA
E-mail: dnt@starpharma.com

Evident Technologies (http://www.evidenttech.com/): The production of quantum dots of various compositions and surface modifications for life science research applications.

Evident Technologies
65 First Street
Troy, NY 12180, USA
E-mail: info@evidenttech.com

Evonik Industries (http://nano.evonik.com/): "Evonik uses nanotechnology to develop innovative products and efficient solutions and to enhance processes. In this way it makes an important contribution to protecting the environment, improving health, and making our lives more comfortable."

Evonik Industries AG
Rellinghauser Straße 1–11
45128 Essen, Germany
E-mail: info@evonik.com

Flamel Technologies (http://www.flamel.com/): Flamel Technologies is a drug delivery company with expertise in polymer chemistry. "Delivery systems for small molecule and protein drugs, providing tailored solutions to the biotech and pharmaceutical industries for optimized controlled release delivery of drugs."

Flamel Technologies
33 avenue du Dr. Georges Levy
69693 Venissieux Cedex, France
E-mail: info@flamel.com

GeneFluidics (http://www.genefluidics.com/): "By integrating novel bio-nano and microfluidic technologies, the Company's revolutionary platform will enable complex tests that are currently performed by skilled technicians in a laboratory to be performed by anyone, anywhere."

GeneFluidics
845 Meridian Street

Irwindale, CA 91010, USA
E-mail: info@GeneFluidics.com

General Electric Healthcare (formerly Amersham Biosciences Corp) (http://www.gehealthcare.com/): A major player in the field on molecular medicine and the utilization of novel nanotechnology applications.

GE Healthcare
800 Centennial Ave.
Piscataway, NJ 08855, USA
E-mail: cs-us@ge.com

ImaRx Therapeutics (http://www.imarx.com/): "The world leader in NanoInvasive™ medicine." ImaRx Therapeutics is utilizing groundbreaking medical technologies to develop products with the potential to revolutionize the treatment of strokes and vascular disease. ImaRx faces near term commercial opportunities in addition to a deep pipeline of development stage compounds.

ImaRx Therapeutics, Inc.
12277 134th NE Suite 202
Redmond, WA 98052, USA
E-mail: imarx@imarx.com

JR Nanotech (http://www.jrnanotech.com/): "Using nano-silver technology to solve age-old healthcare problems."

JR Nanotech
145 Chase Rd.
London
N14 4JP, UK
E-mail: info@jrnanotech.com

Kereos (http://www.kereos.com/): Kereos, Inc. develops targeted molecular imaging agents and therapeutics designed to detect and treat cancer and cardiovascular disease earlier and more specifically than currently possible.

Kereos, Inc.
4041 Forest Park Ave.
Saint Louis, MO 63108, USA
E-mail: info@kereos.com

Keystone Nano (http://www.keystonenano.com/): The production of molecular dots (MD) for the diagnosis and treatment of cancer.

Keystone Nano, Inc.
1981 Pine Hall Rd
State College, PA 16801, USA
E-mail: info@keystonenano.com

KnowmTech (http://www.knowmtech.com/): The development of nanotechnology-based neural networks.

KnowmTech, LLC
117 Bryn Mawr Dr. SE
Albuquerque, NM 87106, USA

Medical Murray (http://www.medicalmurray.com/): "Medical Murray has extensive experience in the injection molding and development of nanoscaled plastic parts."

Medical Murray
400 N Rand Rd.
North Barrington, IL 60010, USA

Mobious Genomics (http://www.mobious.com/): The production of diagnostic and research tools by unifying biological molecular systems and artificial nano-structures.

Mobious Genomics Ltd.
University Innovation Centre
University of Exeter
Rennes Road
Exeter
EX4 4QJ, UK
E-mail: contact@mobious.com

NanoBio® Corporation (http://www.nanobio.com/): "Bio-pharmaceutical company developing and commercializing therapies based on proprietary nanoemulsion technology for the treatment of viral and fungal skin infections and vaginal infections."

NanoBio® Corporation
2311 Green Road, Suite A
Ann Arbor, MI 48105, USA
E-mail: marketing@nanobio.com

NanoBioMagnetics (http://www.nanobmi.com/): "A nano-biomaterials company engaged in the development and commercialization of magnetically responsive nanoparticle technologies (MNP) for a range of human health applications."

NanoBioMagnetics, Inc.
124 N. Bryant Ave.
Edmond, OK 73034, USA
E-mail: nanobio@nanobmi.com

Nanocopoeia (http://www.nanocopeia.com/): "A drug formulation company bringing a proprietary ElectroNanoSpray™ technology for producing nanoparticles to the pharmaceutical and medical device industries."

Nanocopoeia, Inc.
1246 West University Ave.
St. Paul, MN 55104, USA
E-mail: info@nanocopoeia.com

NanoHorizons (http://nanohorizons.com/): "Develop and produce state-of-the-art nanotechnology products and processes for near term biotechnology, pharmaceutical, chemical, and microelectronic applications."

NanoHorizons Inc.
270 Rolling Ridge Drive, Suite 100
Bellefonte, PA 16823, USA
E-mail: info@nanohorizons.com

NanoInk (http://www.nanoink.net/): The use of the Dip Pen Nanolithography™ method for the nano-scale printing of various molecules, including biomolecules, for nanotechnological applications.

NanoInk, Inc.
Illinois Science + Technology Park
8025 Lamon Ave.
Skokie, IL 60077, USA
E-mail: info@nanoink.net

NanoMaterials Ltd. http://www.apnano.com/): NanoMaterials Ltd. is a leading nanotechnology company that develops, manufactures, and markets industrial nano-scale additives for lubricants and enhanced composites.

NanoMaterials, Ltd.
18 Einstein Street,
Weizmann Science Park,
Nes Ziona, 74140, Israel
E-mail: info@apnano.com

Nanomix (http://www.nano.com/): The development of ultrasensitive detection systems based on carbon nanotubes combined with proprietary chemistries.

Nanomix, Inc.
5980 Horton Street
Emeryville, CA 94608, USA
E-mail: info@nano.com

Nanosphere (http://www.nanosphere.us/): "Harnessing the unique properties of matter at the nano-scale in order to commercialize the proprietary chemistry (nanoparticle probes, bio-barcode™ technology, and automated instruments) that is the foundation of its platform."

Nanosphere, Inc.
4088 Commercial Avenue
Northbrook, IL 60062, USA
E-mail: info@nanosphere.us

Nanotherapeutics (http://www.nanotherapeutics.com/): "Nanotherapeutics has developed two proprietary drug delivery technologies, Nanodry™ and Nanocoat™, which produce improved pharmaceuticals at high yield that are substantially more versatile and cost-effective than current technologies."

Nanotherapeutics, Inc.
13859 Progress Blvd., Suite 300
Alachua, FL 32615, USA
E-mail: info@nanotherapeutics.com

Nanoxis (http://www.nanoxis.se/): "A nano-biotechnology company determined to provide generic and optimized tools for membrane protein identification and analysis. Our unique concept is built upon new nanofabrication technologies using soft polymer and fluid-state liquid crystalline materials."

Nanoxis A. B.
MC2 Building A at Chalmers
Kemivägen 9
SE-412 96 Gothenburg, Sweden
E-mail: info@nanoxis.com

Orla Protein Technologies (http://www.orlaproteins.com/): The interface between material science and biology to study the surface of proteins and produce "high density protein arrays, protein-coated particles for therapeutics, bioseparations, surfaces for the attachment and modulation of cells, implantable devices and nanoscale diagnostics".

Orla Protein Technologies Ltd.
Nanotechnology Centre
Newcastle Upon Tyne
NE1 4EP, UK
E-mail: enquiries@orlaproteins.com

Platypus Technologies (http://www.platypustech.com/): "Platypus Technologies, LLC develops, produces and markets nanotechnologies for the life sciences. We produce a variety of nano-structured surfaces for use in research and are also developing a range of products that derive from a proprietary platform technology using liquid crystals for the rapid detection of molecular interactions."

Platypus Technologies, LLC
5520 Nobel Dr., Suite 100
Madison, WI 53711, USA
E-mail: info@platypustech.com

Quantum Dot Corp (presently part of Invitrogen, a subsidiary of Life Technologies) (www.invitrogen.com): The production of quantum dots of various composition and surface modifications for life science research applications.

Life Technologies
3175 Staley Road
Grand Island, NY 14072, USA
E-mail: customerservice@lifetech.com

Schoeller Textil (http://www.nano-sphere.ch): The production of self-cleaning clothes. "The NanoSphere® finishing technology is based on the natural self-cleaning principle and is nearly a perfect copy of nature."

Schoeller Textil AG
Bahnhofstrasse 17
CH-9475 Sevelen, Switzerland
E-mail: info@nano-sphere.ch

Starpharma (http://www.starpharma.com): The use of dendrimer nanotechnology for "the development of high-value dendrimer nanodrugs to address unmet market needs".

Starpharma Holdings Ltd.
75 Commercial Road
Melbourne VIC 3004, Australia
E-mail: info@starpharma.com

Velbionanotech (http://www.velbionanotech.com/): "VBN is dedicated to furthering the art, science and practice of nanotechnology, where biology, chemistry, physics, and mechanical design converge at molecular scale."

Velbionanotech
City Point, Infantry Road,
Bangalore-560 001, India
E-mail: info@velbionanotech.com

Glossary

Actin filament: A two-stranded helical polymer with a diameter of about 7 nm which serves as a major protein component of the cytoskeleton and striated muscles. Also known as *microfilaments*. See *Myosin, Polymer*.

Amino acid: The building blocks of proteins and peptides. A typical amino acid is composed of a chiral carbon linked to an amino group, carboxyl group, and a functional side chain.

Amphiphilic or **Amphipathic:** A chemical compound that has both hydrophilic and hydrophobic nature (from the Greek *amphi*: both, and *philia*: love).

Amyloid fibril: An ordered 7–10 nm protein or peptide fibril that is associated with human disease.

Angstrom (Å): One-tenth of a *Nanometer*.

Archaea or **Archeabacteria:** A branch of prokaryotes that is different from bacteria in many parameters; believed to be a third primary biological kingdom besides bacteria and eukaryotes.

Aromatic compound: A compound which contains a cyclic carbon moiety that includes shared resonant electrons.

Avidin: A glycoprotein that has a very strong affinity for biotin with a dissociation constant to about 10^{-15} M^{-1}.

Atomic force microscope (AFM): A type of scanning probe microscope, with very high-resolution. AFM serves for imaging, measuring, and manipulating matter at the nano-scale.

Bacteriophage: A virus which infects bacteria and replicates in them (from bacteria and the Greek *phagein*: to eat).

Bacterium (*pl.* bacteria): A unicellular prokaryote microorganism that is classified as a lower form of life.

Biomineralization: A process by which organisms produce minerals, often to harden or stiffen existing tissues.

Bionanotechnology: The use of biological principles and building blocks for nanotechnological applications.

Biosensor: A device that combines a biological detection component together with a transducer component for the electrical or optical detection of analytes.

Biotechnology: The technological application of biology in the field of medicine and agriculture.

Biotin: A small organic compound of egg also known as vitamin H or B7 that forms a very strong complex with avidin.

Bottom-up: A process that is based on the formation of complex structures by the coordinated assembly of simple building blocks. See *Top-down*.

Cancer: A class of diseases or disorders that is characterized by the uncontrolled division of cells and formation of metastases.

Composite material: An engineered material that is composed of two or more constituent materials with significantly different physical or chemical properties and which remain separate and distinct within the finished structure.

Contrast agent: An agent that increases the sensitivity of a given imaging technique by improving the noise to signal ratio.

Copolymer: A polymer formed by two or more different types of monomer that are linked in the same chain.

Covalent bond: A chemical bond that is characterized by the sharing of one or more electrons between two atoms.

DNA: Deoxyribonucleic acid, a nucleic acid which contains the information for the synthesis of RNA molecules that is in most cases translated into proteins.

Double helix: A supramolecular structure composed of two congruent helices with the same axis, differing by a translation along the axis. DNA has a double helix structure.

Electroless deposition: A method to reduce metal ions into element metal by the use of chemical reducing agents.

Electron microscope (EM): A type of microscope that uses electrons instead of photons to create an image of the target. The short wavelength of the electron beam allows nanometric resolution compared with hundreds of nanometers resolution using optical microscopy.

Focused ion beam (FIB): An instrument that uses a focused beam of ions (usually gallium ions) for imaging and lithography at nano-scale resolution.

Graphene: a single layer of carbon, just one atom thick.

Graphite: Two-dimensional flat sheets of carbon (from the Greek *graphein*: to draw).

Homology (in its biochemical context): The sharing of a high degree of sequence identity or similarity in the DNA or protein levels.

Hydrogel: A network of polymer chains which contains predominantly water (typically more than 99%). Many hydrogels show nano-scale order.

Hydrophilic: A polar chemical compound that prefers polar solvent such as water (from the Greek *hydro*: water and *philia*: love). See *Amphiphilic*.

Hydrophobic: A non-polar chemical compound which is repelled from a mass of water and prefers non-polar solvents (from the Greek *hydro*: water and *phobos*: fear); sometimes known as "lipophilic."

Inorganic: A chemical compound that does not contain carbon.

Kinesin: A class of motor protein that moves along the microtubules to transport cellular cargo. See *Microtubule*.

Lab-on-a-chip: A device that is capable of handling extremely small fluid volumes down to less than pico-liters for the chemical analysis of analytes.

Lipophilic: See *Hydrophobic*.

Liposome: A spherical phospholipid membrane vesicle with a diameter of tens to hundreds of nm.

Lithography: In general, a method for printing on a smooth surface. In the context of micro- and nano-electronics, it is a method for the patterning of substrates using a mask and source of radiation (that could be photonic, electronic, or ionic).

Microtubule: A protein nano-fiber with a diameter of about 25 nm and length varying from several micrometers to millimeters in axons of nerve cells.

Molar: A concentration unit. Each molar is composed of one mole ($\sim 6 \times 10^{23}$, Avogadro's number) of atoms of molecules in one liter of solvent.

Mole: See *Molar*.

Molecular biology: The study of biology at the level of molecules.

Monomer: A small molecule that could be chemically bonded to other monomers to form a polymer.

Myosin: A motor protein found in eukaryotic tissues that moves along the actin filaments. See *Actin filaments.*

Nanobiotechnology: The use of nanotechnology for biological and medical applications.

Nanometer (*abbr.* nm): 1 billionth or 10^{-9} meter.

Nucleic acid: Polymers composed of nucleotides, either DNA or RNA. See *DNA, Nucleotide, RNA.*

Nucleotide: The main constitute of DNA and RNA, a chemical compound that consists of a heterocyclic base, a sugar, and one or more phosphate groups.

Peptide: Short polymer composed of two or more amino acids. See *Protein.*

Peptide nucleic acid (PNA): A polymer similar to DNA or RNA but differing in the presence of an amide backbone.

Phospholipid: A class of lipids that contain a negatively charged phosphate group. The main constitute of biological membranes.

Photon: The elementary particle responsible for electromagnetic phenomena.

Picomolar: A concentration of 10^{-12} molar.

Polymer: A large molecule consisting of repeating structural units, or monomers, connected by covalent chemical bonds. See *Covalent bond.*

Polysaccharide: A polymer composed of monosaccharides joined together by glycosidic links.

Protein: A long polymer composed of 40–50 amino acids or more. Large proteins can contain thousands of amino acids. See *Peptide*.

Quantum dot: A semiconductor nanostructure that has unique optical and fluorescent properties.

Ribosome: An organelle in cells composed of RNA and proteins that allows the synthesis of proteins.

RNA: Ribonucleic acid, a nucleic acid polymer consisting of nucleotide monomers. mRNA is transcribed from the DNA to serve as the code for the synthesis of proteins. RNA can also serve as a structural and regulatory component.

S-layer: A cell membrane structure composed of proteins and glycoproteins that is found in bacteria and archaea.

Small unilamellar vesicle (SUV): See *Liposome*.

Supramolecular chemistry: A field of chemistry which is concerned with the formation of non-covalent chemical complexes, supramolecules.

Tissue engineering: The ability to engineer biological systems at the level of a tissue rather than cellular or subcellular.

Top-down: A process that is based on the miniaturization of a complex system by the sizing-down of its components. See *Bottom-up*.

Virus: A parasite composed of DNA or RNA molecules that are wrapped in a protein capsid or lipid envelope. See *Bacteriophage*.

Bibliography

Addadi, L. and Weiner, S. (1992) Control and design principles in biological mineralization. *Angew. Chem. Int. Ed.* **31**, 153–169.

Adler-Abramovich, L., Aronov, D., Beker, P., Yevnin, M., Stempler, S., Buzhansky, L., Rosenman, G., and Gazit, E. (2009) Self-assembled arrays of peptide nanotubes by vapour deposition. *Nat. Nanotechnol.* **4**, 849–854.

Adler-Abramovich, L., Badihi-Mossberg, M., Gazit, E., and Rishpon, J. (2010a) Characterization of peptide-nanostructure-modified electrodes and their application for ultrasensitive environmental monitoring. *Small* **6**, 825–831.

Adler-Abramovich, L., Kol, N., Yanai, I., Barlam, D., Shneck, R. Z., Gazit, E., and Rousso, I. (2010b) Self-assembled organic nanostructures with metallic-like stiffness. *Angew. Chem. Int. Ed.* **49**, 9939–9942.

Aggeli, A., Bell, M., Boden, N., Keen, J. N., Knowles, P. F., McLeish, T. C., Pitkeathly, M., and Radford, S. E. (1997) Responsive gels formed by the spontaneous self-assembly of peptides into polymeric beta-sheet tapes. *Nature* **386**, 259–262.

Aili, D. and Stevens, M. M. (2010) Bioresponsive peptide-inorganic hybrid nanomaterials. *Chem. Soc. Rev.* **39**, 3358–3370.

Aizenberg, J., Sundar, V. C., Yablon, A. D., Weaver, J. C., and Chen, G. (2004) Biological glass fibers: Correlation between optical and structural properties. *Proc. Natl. Acad. Sci. USA* **101**, 3358–3363.

Aizenberg, J., Weaver, J. C., Thanawala, M. S., Sundar, V. C., Morse, D. E., and Fratzl, P. (2005) Skeleton of Euplectella *sp.*: Structural hierarchy from the nanoscale to the macroscale. *Science* **309**, 275–278.

Altman, M., Lee, P., Rich, A., and Zhang, S. (2000) Conformational behavior of ionic self-complementary peptides. *Protein Sci.* **9**, 1095–1105.

Altunbas, A., Sharma, N., Lamm, M. S., Yan, C. Q., Nagarkar, R. P., Schneider, J. P., and Pochan, D. J. (2010) Peptide-silica hybrid networks: Biomimetic control of network mechanical behavior. *ACS Nano* **4**, 181–188.

Aniagyei, S. E., DuFort, C., Kao, C. C., and Dragnea, B. (2008) Self-assembly approaches to nanomaterial encapsulation in viral protein cages. *J. Mater. Chem.* **18**, 3763–3774.

Bae, S., Kim, H., Lee, Y., Xu, X. F., Park, J. S., Zheng, Y., Balakrishnan, J., Lei, T., Kim, H. R., Song, Y. I., Kim, Y. J., Kim, K. S., Ozyilmaz, B., Ahn, J. H., Hong, B. H., and Iijima, S. (2010) Roll-to-roll production of 30-inch graphene films for transparent electrodes. *Nat. Nanotechnol.* **5**, 574–578.

Balasubramanian, K. and Burghard, M. (2006) Biosensors based on carbon nanotubes. *Anal. Bioanal. Chem.* **385**, 452–468.

Banerjee, I. A., Yu, L., and Matsui, H. (2003) Cu nanocrystal growth on peptide nanotubes by biomineralization: Size control of Cu nanocrystals by tuning peptide conformation. *Proc. Natl. Acad. Sci. USA* **100**, 14678–14682.

Banwell, E. F., Abelardo, E. S., Adams, D. J., Birchall, M. A., Corrigan, A., Donald, A. M., Kirkland, M., Serpell, L. C., Butler, M. F., and Woolfson, D. N. (2009) Rational design and application of responsive alpha-helical peptide hydrogels. *Nat. Mater.* **8**, 596–600.

Baughman, R. H., Zakhidov, A. A., and de Heer, W. A. (2002) Carbon nanotubes — the route toward applications. *Science* **297**, 787–792.

Baxa, U., Taylor, K. L., Wall, J. S., Simon, M. N., Cheng, N. Q., Wickner, R. B., and Steven, A. C. (2003) Architecture of Ure2p prion filaments — The N-terminal domains form a central core fiber. *J. Biol. Chem.* **278**, 43717–43727.

Bhumiratana, S., Grayson, W. L., Castaneda, A., Rockwood, D. N., Gil, E. S., Kaplan, D. L., and Vunjak-Novakovic, G. (2011) Nucleation and growth of mineralized bone matrix on silk-hydroxyapatite composite scaffolds. *Biomaterials* **32**, 2812–2820.

Bini, E., Knight, D. P., and Kaplan, D. L. (2004) Mapping domain structures in silks from insects and spiders related to protein assembly. *J. Mol. Biol.* **335**, 27–40.

Binnig, G., Rohrer, H., Gerber, Ch., and Weibel, E. (1982) Surface studies by scanning tunneling microscopy. *Phys. Rev. Lett.* **49**, 57–61.

Bong, D. T., Clark, D. T., Granja, J. R., and Ghadiri, M. R. (2001) Self-assembling organic nanotubes. *Angew. Chem. Int. Ed.* **40**, 988–1011.

Branco, M. C. and Schneider, J. P. (2009) Self-assembling materials for therapeutic delivery. *Acta Biomater.* **5**, 817–831.

Braun, E., Eichen, Y., Sivan, U., and Ben-Yoseph, G. (1998) DNA-templated assembly and electrode attachment of a conducting silver wire. *Nature* **391**, 775–778.

Briones, C. and Moreno, M. (2012) Applications of peptide nucleic acids (PNAs) and locked nucleic acids (LNAs) in biosensor development. *Anal. Bioanal. Chem.* **402**, 3071–3089.

Brott, L. L., Naik, R. R., Pikas, D. J., Kirkpatrick, S. M., Tomlin, D. W., Whitlock, P. W., Clarson, S. J., and Stone, M. O. (2001) Ultrafast holographic nanopatterning of biocatalytically formed silica. *Nature* **413**, 291–293.

Brutchey, R. L. and Morse, D. E. (2008) Silicatein and the translation of its molecular mechanism of biosilicification into low temperature nanomaterial synthesis. *Chem. Rev.* **108**, 4915–4934.

Bull, S. R., Guler, M. O., Bras, R. E., Meade, T. J., and Stupp, S. I. (2005) Self-assembled peptide amphiphile nanofibers conjugated to MRI contrast agents. *Nano Lett.* **5**, 1–4.

Caldorera-Moore, M. E., Liechty, W. B., and Peppas, N. A. (2011) Responsive theranostic systems: Integration of diagnostic imaging agents and responsive controlled release drug delivery carriers. *Acc. Chem. Res.* **44**, 1061–1070.

Carny, O., Shalev, D. E., and Gazit, E. (2006) Fabrication of coaxial metal nanocables using a self-assembled peptide nanotube scaffold. *Nano Lett.* **6**, 1594–1597.

Castillo, J., Dimaki, M., and Svendsen, W. E. (2009) Manipulation of biological samples using micro and nano techniques. *Integr. Biol.* **1**, 30–42.

Cha, J. N., Shimizu, K., Zhou, Y., Christiansen, S. C., Chmelka, B. F., Stucky, G. D., and Morse, D. E. (1999) Silicatein filaments and subunits from a marine sponge direct the polymerization of silica and silicones *in vitro*. *Proc. Natl. Acad. Sci. USA* **96**, 361–365.

Chapman, M. R., Robinson, L. S., Pinkner, J. S., Roth, R., Heuser, J., Hammar, M., Normark, S., and Hulgren, S. J. (2002) Role of *Escherichia coli* curli operons in directing amyloid fiber formation. *Science* **295**, 851–855.

Charalambidis, G., Kasotakis, E., Lazarides, T., Mitraki, A., and Coutsolelos, A. G. (2011) Self-assembly into spheres of a hybrid diphenylalanine-porphyrin: Increased fluorescence lifetime and conserved electronic properties. *Chemistry* **17**, 7213–7219.

Chen, C., Daniel, M. C., Quinkert, Z. T., De, M., Stein, B., Bowman, V. D., Chipman, P. R., Rotello, V. M., Kao, C. C., and Dragnea, B. (2006) Nanoparticle-templated assembly of viral protein cages. *Nano Lett.* **6**, 611–615.

Cole, L. A. (1997) Immunoassay of human chorionic gonadotropin, its free sub-units, and metabolites. *Clin. Chem.* **43**, 2233–2243.

Collier, J. H., Rudra, J. S., Gasiorowski, J. Z., and Jung, J. P. (2010) Multi-component extracellular matrices based on peptide self-assembly. *Chem. Soc. Rev.* **39**, 3413–3424.

Collins, P. G., Arnold, M. S., and Avouris, P. (2001) Engineering carbon nano-tubes and nanotube circuits using electrical breakdown. *Science* **292**, 706–709.

Cui, H. G., Webber, M. J., and Stupp, S. I. (2010) Self-assembly of peptide amphiphiles: From molecules to nanostructures to biomaterials. *Biopolymers* **94**, 1–18.

Das, R., Kiley, P. J., Segal, M., Norville, J., Yu, A. A., Wang, L. Y., Trammell, S. A., Reddick, L. E., Kumar, R., Stellacci, F., Lebedev, N., Schnur, J., Bruce, B. D., Zhang, S. G., and Baldo, M. (2004) Integration of photosynthetic protein molecular complexes in solid-state electronic devices. *Nano Lett.* **4**, 1079–1083.

de la Rica, R., Mendoza, E., Lechuga, L. M., and Matsui, H. (2008) Label-free pathogen detection with sensor chips assembled from peptide nanotubes. *Angew. Chem. Int. Ed.* **47**, 9752–9755.

de la Rica, R., Pejoux, C., and Matsui, H. (2011) Assemblies of functional pep-tides and their applications in building blocks for biosensors. *Adv. Funct. Mater.* **21**, 1018–1026.

DeLong, E. F., and Pace, N. R. (2001) Environmental diversity of bacteria and archaea. *Syst. Biol.* **50**, 470–478.

de Pablo, P. J., Schaap, I. A., MacKintosh, F. C., and Schmidt, C. F. (2003) Deformation and collapse of microtubules on the nanometer scale. *Phys. Rev. Lett.* **91**, 098101.

Dickerson, M. B., Naik, R. R., Stone, M. O., Cai, Y., and Sandhage, K. H. (2004) Identification of peptides that promote the rapid precipitation of germania nanoparticle networks via use of a peptide display library. *Chem. Commun.* **15**, 1776–1777.

Dinca, V., Kasotakis, E., Catherine, J., Mourka, A., Ranella, A., Ovsianikov, A., Chichkov, B. N., Farsari, M., Mitraki, A., and Fotakis, C. (2008) Directed three-dimensional patterning of self-assembled peptide fibrils. *Nano Lett.* **8**, 538–543.

Djalali, R., Chen, Y. F., and Matsui, H. (2003) Au nanocrystal growth on nanotubes controlled by conformations and charges of sequenced peptide templates. *J. Am. Chem. Soc.* **125**, 5873–5879.

Douglas, T. (2003) Materials science. A bright bio-inspired future. *Science* **299**, 1192–1193.

Douglas, T., Strable, E., Willits, D., Aitouchen, A., Libera, M., and Young, M. (2002) Protein engineering of a viral cage for constrained nanomaterials synthesis. *Adv. Mater.* **4**, 415–418.

Drakakis, T. S., Papadakis, G., Sambani, K., Filippidis, G., Georgiou, S., Gizeli, E., Fotakis, C., and Farsari, M. (2006) Construction of three-dimensional biomolecule structures employing femtosecond lasers. *Appl. Phys. Lett.* **89**, 3.

Drexler, E. K. (1981) Molecular engineering: An approach to the development of general capabilities for molecular manipulation. *Proc. Natl. Acad. Sci. USA* **78**, 5275–5278.

Drexler, E. K. (1986) *Engines of Creation: The Coming Era of Nanotechnology.* Anchor Books/Doubleday, New York. (Also available online: http://e-drexler.com/p/06/00/EOC_Cover.html.)

Drexler, E. K. (1992) *Nanosystems: Molecular Machinery, Manufacturing, and Computation.* Wiley Interscience, New York.

Dujardin, E., Peet, C., Stubbs, G., Culver, J. N., and Mann, S. (2003) Organization of metallic nanoparticles using tobacco mosaic virus templates. *Nano Lett.* **3**, 413–417.

Eigler, D. M. and Schweizer, E. K. (1990) Positioning single atoms with a scanning tunneling microscope. *Nature* **344**, 524–526.

Eisoldt, L., Smith, A., and Scheibel, T. (2011) Decoding the secrets of spider silk. *Mater. Today* **14**, 80–86.

Eisoldt, L., Thamm, C., and Scheibel, T. (2012) Review the role of terminal domains during storage and assembly of spider silk proteins. *Biopolymers* **97**, 355–361.

Elliot, M. A., Karoonuthaisiri, N., Huang, J., Bibb, M. J., Cohen, S. N., Kao, C. M., and Buttner, M. J. (2003) The chaplins: A family of hydrophobic cell-surface proteins involved in aerial mycelium formation in *Streptomyces coelicolor.* *Genes Dev.* **17**, 1727–1740.

Ellis-Behnke, R. G., Liang, Y. X., You, S. W., Tay, D. K. C., Zhang, S. G., So, K. F., and Schneider, G. E. (2006) Nano neuro knitting: Peptide nanofiber scaffold for brain repair and axon regeneration with functional return of vision. *Proc. Natl. Acad. Sci. USA* **103**, 5054–5059.

Empedocles, S. A. and Bawendi, M. G. (1997) Quantum-confined stark effect in single CdSe nanocrystallite quantum dots. *Science* **278**, 2114–2117.

Espinosa, H. D., Rim, J. E., Barthelat, F., and Buehler, M. J. (2009) Merger of structure and material in nacre and bone — perspectives on *de novo* biomimetic materials. *Prog. Mater. Sci.* **54**, 1059–1100.

Feldkamp, U. and Niemeyer, C. M. (2006) Rational design of DNA nanoarchitectures. *Angew. Chem. Int. Ed.* **45**, 1856–1876.

Fisher, O. Z., Khademhosseini, A., Langer, R., and Peppas, N. A. (2010) Bioinspired materials for controlling stem cell fate. *Acc. Chem. Res.* **43**, 419–428.

Foley, J., Schmid, H., Stutz, R., and Delamarche, E. (2005) Microcontact printing of proteins inside microstructures. *Langmuir* **21**, 11296–11303.

Fowler, D. M., Koulov, A. V., Alory-Jost, C., Marks, M. S., Balch, W. E., and Kelly, J. W. (2006) Functional amyloid formation within mammalian tissue. *PLOS Biol.* **4**, 100–107.

Fowler, D. M., Koulov, A. V., Balch, W. E., and Kelly, J. W. (2007) Functional amyloid — from bacteria to humans. *Trends Biochem. Sci.* **32**, 217–224.

Fraenkel-Conrat, H., Singer, B., and Williams, R. C. (1957) Infectivity of viral nucleic acid. *Biochim. Biophys. Acta* **25**, 87–96.

Fratzl, P. and Weinkamer, R. (2007) Nature's hierarchical materials. *Prog. Mater. Sci.* **52**, 1263–1334.

Freestone, I., Meeks, N., Sax, M., and Higgitt, C. (2007) The Lycurgus Cup — A Roman nanotechnology. *Gold Bull.* **40**, 270–277.

Fromherz, P. (2002) Electrical interfacing of nerve cells and semiconductor chips. *ChemPhysChem* **3**, 276–284.

Garner, M. M. and Rau, D. C. (1995) Water release associated with specific binding of gal repressor. *EMBO J.* **14**, 1257–1263.

Gazit, E. (2002a) A possible role for pi-stacking in the self-assembly of amyloid fibrils. *FASEB J.* **16**, 77–83.

Gazit, E. (2002b) Mechanistic studies of the process of amyloid fibrils formation by the use of peptide fragments and analogues: Implications for the design of fibrillization inhibitors. *Curr. Med. Chem.* **9**, 1725–1735.

Gazit, E. (2007) Use of biomolecular templates for the fabrication of metal nanowires. *Febs J.* **274**, 317–322.

Geddes, A. J., Parker, K. D., Atkins, E. D. T., and Beighton, A. (1968) "Cross-beta" conformation in proteins. *J. Mol. Biol.* **32**, 343–358.

Geim, A. K. (2009) Graphene: Status and prospects. *Science* **324**, 1530–1534.

Gelain, F., Horii, A., and Zhang, S. G. (2007) Designer self-assembling peptide scaffolds for 3-D tissue cell cultures and regenerative medicine. *Macromol. Biosci.* **7**, 544–551.

Ghadiri, M. R., Granja, J. R., Milligan, R. A., McRee, D. E., and Khazanovich, N. (1993) Self-assembling organic nanotubes based on a cyclic peptide architecture. *Nature* **366**, 324–347.

Ghadiri, M. R., Granja, J. R., and Buehler, L. K. (1994) Artificial transmembrane ion channels from self-assembling peptide nanotubes. *Nature* **369**, 301–304.

Gilead, S. and Gazit, E. (2005) Self-organization of short peptide fragments: From amyloid fibrils to nanoscale supramolecular assemblies. *Supramol. Chem.* **17**, 87–92.

Goel, A., Howard, J. B., and Sande, J. B. V. (2004) Size analysis of single fullerene molecules by electron microscopy. *Carbon* **42**, 1907–1915.

Gratzel, M. (2009) Recent advances in sensitized mesoscopic solar cells. *Acc. Chem. Res.* **42**, 1788–1798.

Greenwald, J. and Riek, R. (2010) Biology of amyloid: Structure, function, and regulation. *Structure* **18**, 1244–1260.

Gungormus, M., Branco, M., Fong, H., Schneider, J. P., Tamerler, C., and Sarikaya, M. (2010) Self assembled bi-functional peptide hydrogels with biomineralization-directing peptides. *Biomaterials* **31**, 7266–7274.

Gyorvary, E., Schroedter, A., Talapin, D. V., Weller, H., Pum, D., and Sleytr, U. B. (2004) Formation of nanoparticle arrays on S-layer protein lattices. *J. Nanosci. Nanotechnol.* **4**, 115–120.

Haines-Butterick, L., Rajagopal, K., Branco, M., Salick, D., Rughani, R., Pilarz, M., Lamm, M. S., Pochan, D. J., and Schneider, J. P. (2007) Controlling hydrogelation kinetics by peptide design for three-dimensional encapsulation and injectable delivery of cells. *Proc. Natl. Acad. Sci. USA* **104**, 7791–7796.

Hamada, D., Yanagihara, I., and Tsumoto, K. (2004) Engineering amyloidogenicity towards the development of nanofibrillar materials. *Trends Biotechnol.* **22**, 93–97.

Hart, S. L. (2005) Lipid carriers for gene therapy. *Curr. Drug Deliv.* **2**, 423–428.

Hartgerink, J. D. Beniash, E., and Stupp, S. I. (2001) Self-assembly and mineralization of peptide-amphiphile nanofibers. *Science* **294**, 1684–1688.

Hauser, C. A. E. and Zhang, S. G. (2010) Designer self-assembling peptide nanofiber biological materials. *Chem. Soc. Rev.* **39**, 2780–2790.

Holmes, T. C., de Lacalle, S., Su, X., Liu, G., Rich, A., and Zhang, S. (2000) Extensive neurite outgrowth and active synapse formation on self-assembling peptide scaffolds. *Proc. Natl. Acad. Sci. USA* **97**, 6728–6733.

Horii, A., Wang, X. M., Gelain, F., and Zhang, S. G. (2007) Biological designer self-assembling peptide nanofiber scaffolds significantly enhance osteoblast proliferation, differentiation and 3-D migration. *PLOS ONE* **2**, 9.

Horne, W. S., Ashkenasy, N., and Ghadiri, M. R. (2005) Modulating charge transfer through cyclic D, L-alpha-peptide self-assembly. *Chemistry* **11**, 1137–1144.

Hunter, C. A. (1993) Arene-Arene Interactions: Electrostatic or charge transfer. *Angew. Chem. Int. Ed.* **32**, 1584–1586.

Iconomidou, V. A. and Hamodrakas, S. J. (2008) Natural protective amyloids. *Curr. Protein Pept. Sci.* **9**, 291–309.

Iijima, S. (1991) Helical microtubules of graphitic carbon. *Nature* **354**, 56–58.

Ilk, N., Egelseer, E. M., and Sleytr, U. W. (2011) S-layer fusion proteins-construction principles and applications. *Curr. Opin. Biotechnol.* **22**, 824–831.

Jaffari, S. A. and Turner, A. P. (1995) Recent advances in amperometric glucose biosensors for *in vivo* monitoring. *Physiol. Meas.* **16**, 1–15.

Jaremko, J. and Rorstad, O. (1998) Advances toward the implantable artificial pancreas for treatment of diabetes. *Diabetes Care* **21**, 444–450.

Jarrett, J. T. and Lansbury, P. T. Jr. (1993) Seeding "one-dimensional crystallization" of amyloid: A pathogenic mechanism in Alzheimer's disease and scrapie? *Cell* **73**, 1055–1058.

Jin, H.-J. and Kaplan, D. E. (2003) Mechanism of silk processing in insects and spiders. *Nature* **424**, 1057–1061.

Jin, S., Hu, Y. X., Gu, Z. J., Liu, L., and Wu, H. C. (2011) Application of quantum dots in biological imaging. *J. Nanomater.* **2011**, Article ID 834139, 13 pages.

Kacar, T., Zin, M. T., So, C., Wilson, B., Ma, H., Gul-Karaguler, N., Jen, A. K. Y., Sarikaya, M., and Tamerler, C. (2009) Directed self-immobilization of alkaline phosphatase on micro-patterned substrates via genetically fused metal-binding peptide. *Biotechnol. Bioeng.* **103**, 696–705.

Kamiya, S., Minamikawa, H., Jung, J. H., Yang, B., Masuda, M., and Shimizu, T. (2005) Molecular structure of glucopyranosylamide lipid and nanotube morphology. *Langmuir* **21**, 743–750.

Kane, R. S., Takayama, S., Ostuni, E., Ingber, D. E., and Whitesides, G. M. (1999) Patterning proteins and cells using soft lithography. *Biomaterials* **20**, 2363–2376.

Kasotakis, E., Mossou, E., Adler-Abramovich, L., Mitchell, E. P., Forsyth, V. T., Gazit, E., and Mitraki, A. (2009) Design of metal-binding sites onto self-assembled peptide fibrils. *Biopolymers* **92**, 164–172.

Katz, E. and Willner, I. (2004) Biomolecule-functionalized carbon nanotubes: Applications in nanobioelectronics. *ChemPhysChem* **5**, 1084–1104.

Kaul, R. A., Syed, N. I., and Fromherz, P. (2004) Neuron-semiconductor chip with chemical synapse between identified neurons. *Phys. Rev. Lett.* **92**, 038102.

Keren, K., Krueger, M., Gilad, R., Ben-Yoseph, G., Sivan, U., and Braun, E. (2002) Sequence-specific molecular lithography on single DNA molecules. *Science* **297**, 72–75.

Khatayevich, D., Gungormus, M., Yazici, H., So, C., Cetinel, S., Ma, H., Jen, A., Tamerler, C., and Sarikaya, M. (2010) Biofunctionalization of materials for implants using engineered peptides. *Acta Biomater.* **6**, 4634–4641.

Kiley, P., Zhao, X., Vaughn, M., Baldo, M. A., Bruce, B. D., and Zhang, S. (2005) Self-assembling peptide detergents stabilize isolated photosystem I on a dry surface for an extended time. *PLOS Biol.* **3**, e230.

Kim, J. H., Lee, M., Lee, J. S., and Park, C. B. (2012) Self-assembled light-harvesting peptide nanotubes for mimicking natural photosynthesis. *Angew. Chem. Int. Ed.* **51**, 517–520.

King, C. Y., Tittmann, P., Gross, H., Gebert, R., Aebi, M., and Wuthrich, K. (1997). Prion-inducing domain 2–114 of yeast Sup35 protein transforms *in vitro* into amyloid-like filaments. *Proc. Natl. Acad. Sci. USA* **94**, 6618–6622.

Kirkham, J., Firth, A., Vernals, D., Boden, N., Robinson, C., Shore, R. C., Brookes, S. J., and Aggeli, A. (2007) Self-assembling peptide scaffolds promote enamel remineralization. *J. Dent. Res.* **86**, 426–430.

Kisailus, D., Choi, J. H., Weaver, J. C., Yang, W. J., and Morse, D. E. (2005) Enzymatic synthesis and nanostructural control of gallium oxide at low temperature. *Adv. Mater.* **17**, 314–318.

Kisiday, J., Jin, M., Kurz, B., Hung, H., Semino, C., Zhang, S., and Grodzinsky, A. J. (2002) Self-assembling peptide hydrogel fosters chondrocyte extracellular matrix production and cell division: Implications for cartilage tissue repair. *Proc. Natl. Acad. Sci. USA* **99**, 9996–10001.

Knez, M., Bittner, A. M., Boes, C., Wege, C., Jeske, H., Maiß, K., and Kern, K. (2003). Biotemplate synthesis of 3-nm nickel and cobalt nanowires. *Nano Lett.* **3**, 1079–1082.

Knez, M., Sumser, M. P., Bittner, A. M., Wege, C., Jeske, H., Martin, T. P., and Kern, K. (2004). Spatially selective nucleation of metal clusters on the tobacco mosaic virus. *Adv. Funct. Mat.* **14**, 114–119.

Knowles, T. P. J. and Buehler, M. J. (2011) Nanomechanics of functional and pathological amyloid materials. *Nat. Nanotechnol.* **6**, 469–479.

Kol, N., Abramovich, L., Barlam, D., Shneck, R. Z., Gazit E., and Rousso, I. (2005) Self-assembled peptide nanotubes are uniquely rigid bioinspired supramolecular structures. *Nano Lett.* **5**, 1343–1346.

Kroger, N., Deutzmann, R., and Sumper, M. (1999) Polycationic peptides from diatom biosilica that direct silica nanosphere formation. *Science* **286**, 1129–1132.

Kroto, H. W., Heath, J. R., O'Brien, S. C., Curl, R. F., and Smalley, R. E. (1985) C60: Buckminsterfullerene. *Nature* **318**, 162–163.

Kubik, S. (2002) High-performance fibers from spider silk. *Angew. Chem. Int. Ed.* **41**, 2721–2723.

Kumar, P., Pillay, V., Modi, G., Choonara, Y., du Toit, L., and Naidoo, D. (2011) Self-assembling peptides: Implications for patenting in drug delivery and tissue engineering. *Recent Pat. Drug Deliv. Formul.* **5**, 24–51.

Kumara, M. T., Tripp, B. C., and Muralidharan, S. (2007a) Exciton energy transfer in self-assembled quantum dots on bioengineered bacterial flagella nanotubes. *J. Phys. Chem. C* **111**, 5276–5280.

Kumara, M. T., Tripp, B. C., and Muralidharan, S. (2007b) Self-assembly of metal nanoparticles and nanotubes on bioengineered flagella scaffolds. *Chem. Mater.* **19**, 2056–2064.

Lakshmanan, A., Zhang, S. G., and Hauser, C. A. E. (2012) Short self-assembling peptides as building blocks for modern nanodevices. *Trends Biotechnol.* **30**, 155–165.

Langer, R. (2000) Biomaterials in drug delivery and tissue engineering: One laboratory's experience. *Acc. Chem. Res.* **33**, 94–101.

Larsen, P., Nielsen, J. L., Dueholm, M. S., Wetzel, R., Otzen, D., and Nielsen, P. H. (2007) Amyloid adhesins are abundant in natural biofilms. *Environ. Microbiol.* **9**, 3077–3090.

Lee, J. H., Yigit, M. V., Mazumdar, D., and Lu, Y. (2010) Molecular diagnostic and drug delivery agents based on aptamer-nanomaterial conjugates. *Adv. Drug Deliver. Rev.* **62**, 592–605.

Lee, K.-B., Park, S.-J., Mirkin, C. A., Smith, J. C., and Mrksich, M. (2002) Protein nanoarrays generated by dip-pen nanolithography. *Science* **295**, 1702–1705.

Lee, K.-B., Lim, J.-H., and Mirkin, C. A. (2003) Protein nanostructures formed via direct-write dip-pen nanolithography. *J. Am. Chem. Soc.* **125**, 5588–5589.

Lee, S. W., Mao, C., Flynn, C. E., and Belcher, A. M. (2002) Ordering of quantum dots using genetically engineered viruses. *Science* **296**, 892–895.

Lee, S. Y., Royston, E., Culver, J. N., and Harris, M. T. (2005) Improved metal cluster deposition on a genetically engineered tobacco mosaic virus template. *Nanotechnology* **16**, S435–S441.

Lee, S. Y., Choi, J. W., Royston, E., Janes, D. B., Culver, J. N., and Harris, M. T. (2006) Deposition of platinum clusters on surface-modified tobacco mosaic virus. *J. Nanosci. Nanotechnol.* **6**, 974–981.

Lehn, J. M. (2002) Toward self-organization and complex matter. *Science* **295**, 2400–2403.

Liang, Y. X., Cheung, S. W. H., Chan, K. C. W., Wu, E. X., Tay, D. K. C., and Ellis-Behnke, R. G. (2011) CNS regeneration after chronic injury using a self-assembled nanomaterial and MEMRI for real-time *in vivo* monitoring. *Nanomed.-Nanotechnol.* **7**, 351–359.

Liepold, L. O., Abedin, M. J., Buckhouse, E. D., Frank, J. A., Young, M. J., and Douglas, T. (2009) Supramolecular protein cage composite MR contrast agents with extremely efficient relaxivity properties. *Nano Lett.* **9**, 4520–4526.

Li Jeon, N., Baskaran, H., Dertinger, S. K., Whitesides, G. M., Van de Water, L., and Toner, M. (2002) Neutrophil chemotaxis in linear and complex gradients of interleukin-8 formed in a microfabricated device. *Nat. Biotechnol.* **20**, 826–830.

Liu, H. R., Jin, L., Koh, S. B. S., Atanasov, I., Schein, S., Wu, L., and Zhou, Z. H. (2010) Atomic structure of human adenovirus by cryo-em reveals interactions among protein networks. *Science* **329**, 1038–1043.

Liu, Z., Zhang, D., Han, S., Li, C., Lei, B., Lu, W., Fang, J., and Zhou, C. (2005) Single crystalline magnetite nanotubes. *J. Am. Chem. Soc.* **127**, 6–7.

Loo, Y., Zhang, S. G., and Hauser, C. A. E. (2012) From short peptides to nanofibers to macromolecular assemblies in biomedicine. *Biotechnol. Adv.* **30**, 593–603.

Madhavaiah, C. and Verma, S. (2004) Self-aggregation of reverse bis peptide conjugate derived from the unstructured region of the prion protein. *Chem. Commun.* **21**, 638–639.

Madhavaiah, C. and Verma, S. (2005) Copper-metalated peptide palindrome derived from prion octarepeat: Synthesis, aggregation, and oxidative transformations. *Bioorg. Med. Chem.* **13**, 3241–3248.

Maji, S. K., Schubert, D., Rivier, C., Lee, S., Rivier, J. E., and Riek, R. (2008) Amyloid as a depot for the formulation of long-acting drugs. *PLOS Biol.* **6**, 240–252.

Maji, S. K., Perrin, M. H., Sawaya, M. R., Jessberger, S., Vadodaria, K., Rissman, R. A., Singru, P. S., Nilsson, K. P. R., Simon, R., Schubert, D., Eisenberg, D., Rivier, J., Sawchenko, P., Vale, W., and Riek, R. (2009) Functional amyloids as natural storage of peptide hormones in pituitary secretory granules. *Science* **325**, 328–332.

Mann, S. and Weiner, S. (1999) Biomineralization: Structural questions at all length scales. *J. Struct. Biol.* **126**, 179–181.

Mao, C., Solis, D. J., Reiss, B. D., Kottmann, S. T., Sweeney, R. Y., Hayhurst, A., Georgiou, G., Iverson, B., and Belcher, A. M. (2004) Virus-based toolkit for the directed synthesis of magnetic and semiconducting nanowires. *Science* **303**, 213–217.

Margulis, L., Salitra, G., Tenne, R., and Talianker, M. (1993) Nested fullerene-like structures. *Nature* **365**, 113–114.

Martin, R., Waldmann, L., and Kaplan, D. L. (2003) Supramolecular assembly of collagen triblock peptides. *Biopolymers* **70**, 435–444.

Marx, A., Muller, J., and Mandelkow, E. (2005) The structure of microtubule motor proteins. *Adv. Protein Chem.* **71**, 299–344.

Mathe, J., Aksimentiev, A., Nelson, D. R., Schulten, K., and Meller, A. (2005) Orientation discrimination of single-stranded DNA inside the alpha-hemolysin membrane channel. *Proc. Natl. Acad. Sci. USA* **102**, 12377–12382.

Matson, J. B. and Stupp, S. I. (2012) Self-assembling peptide scaffolds for regenerative medicine. *Chem. Commun.* **48**, 26–33.

Matsui, H., Pan, S., Gologan, B., and Jonas, S. H. (2000) Bolaamphiphile nanotube-templated metallized wires. *J. Phys. Chem. B*, **104**, 9576–9579.

Meller, A., Nivon, L., Brandin, E., Golovchenko, J., and Branton, D. (2000) Rapid nanopore discrimination between single polynucleotide molecules. *Proc. Natl. Acad. Sci. USA* **97**, 1079–1084.

Merrifield, R. B. (1965) Automated synthesis of peptides. *Science* **150**, 178–185.

Mitraki, A. (2010) Protein aggregation: From inclusion bodies to amyloid and biomaterials. *Adv. Protein Chem. Struct. Biol.* **79**, 89–125.

Morais-Cabral, J. H., Lee, A., Cohen, S. L., Chait, B. T., Li, M., and Mackinnon, R. (1998) Crystal structure and functional analysis of the HERG potassium channel N terminus: A eukaryotic PAS domain. *Cell* **95**, 649–655.

Mostaert, A. S., Higgins, M. J., Fukuma, T., Rindi, F., and Jarvis, S. P. (2006) Nanoscale mechanical characterisation of amyloid fibrils discovered in a natural adhesive. *J. Biol. Phys.* **32**, 393–401.

Mostaert, A. S., Giordani, C., Crockett, R., Karsten, U., Schumann, R., and Jarvis, S. P. (2009) Characterisation of amyloid nanostructures in the natural adhesive of unicellular subaerial algae. *J. Adhesion.* **85**, 465–483.

Naik, R. R., Whitlock, P. W., Rodriguez, F., Brott, L. L., Glawe, D. D., Clarson, S. J., and Stone, M. O. (2003) Controlled formation of biosilica structures *in vitro*. *Chem. Commun.* **2003**, 238–239.

Nakashima, N., Asakuma, S., and Kunitake, T. (1985) Optical microscopic study of helical superstructures of chiral bilayer membranes. *J. Am. Chem. Soc.* **107**, 509–510.

Nam, J.-M., Thaxton, C. S., and Mirkin, C. A. (2003) Nanoparticle-based bio-bar codes for the ultrasensitive detection of proteins. *Science* **301**, 1884–1886.

Nam, K. T., Kim, D. W., Yoo, P. J., Chiang, C. Y., Meethong, N., Hammond, P. T., Chiang, Y. M., and Belcher, A. M. (2006) Virus-enabled synthesis and assembly of nanowires for lithium ion battery electrodes. *Science* **312**, 885–888.

Nam, Y. S., Shin, T., Park, H., Magyar, A. P., Choi, K., Fantner, G., Nelson, K. A., and Belcher, A. M. (2010) Virus-templated assembly of porphyrins into light-harvesting nanoantennae. *J. Am. Chem. Soc.* **132**, 1462–1463.

Nelson, R. and Eisenberg, D. (2006) Recent atomic models of amyloid fibril structure. *Curr. Opin. Struct. Biol.* **16**, 260–265.

Ng, E. W. M., Shima, D. T., Calias, P., Cunningham, E. T., Guyer, D. R., and Adamis, A. P. (2006) Pegaptanib, a targeted anti-VEGF aptamer for ocular vascular disease. *Nat. Rev. Drug Discov.* **5**, 123–132.

Nielsen, P. E. (1995) DNA analogues with nonphosphodiester backbones. *Annu. Rev. Biophys. Biomol. Struct.* **24**, 167–183.

Novoselov, K. S., Geim, A. K., Morozov, S. V., Jiang, D., Zhang, Y., Dubonos, S. V., Grigorieva, I. V., and Firsov, A. A. (2004) Electric field effect in atomically thin carbon films. *Science* **306**, 666–669.

Nuraje, N., Banerjee, I. A., MacCuspie, R. I., Yu, L., and Matsui, H. (2004) Biological bottom-up assembly of antibody nanotubes on patterned antigen arrays. *J. Am. Chem. Soc.* **126**, 8088–8089.

Ostrov, N. and Gazit, E. (2010) Genetic engineering of biomolecular scaffolds for the fabrication of organic and metallic nanowires. *Angew. Chem. Int. Ed.* **49**, 3018–3021.

Otzen, D. (2010) Functional amyloid turning swords into plowshares. *Prion* **4**, 256–264.

Ozbas, B., Kretsinger, J., Rajagopal, K., Schneider, J. P., and Pochan, D. J. (2004) Salt-triggered peptide folding and consequent self-assembly into hydrogels with tunable modulus. *Macromolecules* **37**, 7331–7337.

Pandya, M. J., Spooner, G. M., Sunde, M., Thorpe, J. R., Rodger, A., and Woolfson, D. N. (2000) Sticky-end assembly of a designed peptide fiber provides insight into protein fibrillogenesis. *Biochemistry* **39**, 8728–8734.

Parker, M. W. and Feil, S. C. (2005) Pore-forming protein toxins: From structure to function. *Prog. Biophys. Mol. Biol.* **88**, 91–142.

Patolsky, F., Weizmann, Y., and Willner, I. (2004a) Actin-based metallic nanowires as bio-nanotransporters. *Nat. Mater.* **3**, 692–695.

Patolsky, F., Zheng, G., Hayden, O., Lakadamyali, M., Zhuang, X., and Lieber, C. M. (2004b) Electrical detection of single viruses. *Proc. Natl. Acad. Sci USA* **101**, 14017–14022.

Patwardhan, S. V. (2011) Biomimetic and bioinspired silica: Recent developments and applications. *Chem. Commun.* **47**, 7567–7582.

Perry, C. C. and Keeling-Tucker, T. (2000) Biosilicification: The role of the organic matrix in structure control. *J. Biol. Inorg. Chem.* **5**, 537–550.

Pfeffer, R. (1927) *Organische Molekülverbindungen*. Enke, Stuttgart.

Phillips, M. A., Gran, M. L., and Peppas, N. A. (2010) Targeted nanodelivery of drugs and diagnostics. *Nano Today* **5**, 143–159.

Pinheiro, A. V., Han, D. R., Shih, W. M., and Yan, H. (2011) Challenges and opportunities for structural DNA nanotechnology. *Nat. Nanotechnol.* **6**, 763–772.

Pouget, E., Dujardin, E., Cavalier, A., Moreac, A., Valery, C., Marchi-Artzner, V., Weiss, T., Renault, A., Paternostre, M., and Artzner, F. (2007) Hierarchical architectures by synergy between dynamical template self-assembly and biomineralization. *Nature Mater.* **6**, 434–439.

Pum, D., Neubauer, A., Gyorvary, E., Sara, M., and Sleytr, U. B. (2000) S-layer proteins as basic building blocks in a biomolecular construction kit. *Nanotechnology* **11**, 100–107.

Reches, M. and Gazit, E. (2003) Casting metal nanowires within discrete self-assembled peptide nanotubes. *Science* **300**, 625–627.

Reches, M. and Gazit, E. (2004) Formation of closed-cage nanostructures by self-assembly of aromatic dipeptides. *Nano Lett.* **4**, 581–585.

Reches, M. and Gazit, E. (2005) Self-assembly of peptide nanotubes and amyloid-like structures by charged-termini capped diphenylalanine peptide analogues. *Israel J. Chem.* **45**, 363–371.

Reches, M. and Gazit, E. (2006a) Molecular self-assembly of peptide nanostructures: Mechanism of association and potential uses. *Curr. Nanoscience* **2**, 105–111.

Reches, M. and Gazit, E. (2006b) Controlled patterning of aligned self-assembled peptide nanotubes. *Nat. Nanotechnol.* **1**, 195–200.

Reddy, V. S., Natchiar, S. K., Stewart, P. L., and Nemerow, G. R. (2010) Crystal structure of human adenovirus at 3.5 angstrom resolution. *Science* **329**, 1071–1075.

Rothemund, P. W. K. (2006) Folding DNA to create nanoscale shapes and patterns. *Nature* **440**, 297–302.

Ryadnov, M. G., Bella, A., Timson, S., and Woolfson, D. N. (2009) Modular design of peptide fibrillar nano- to microstructures. *J. Am. Chem. Soc.* **131**, 13240–13241.

Sacca, B. and Niemeyer, C. M. (2012) DNA origami: The art of folding DNA. *Angew. Chem. Int. Ed.* **51**, 58–66.

Sawaya, M. R., Sambashivan, S., Nelson, R., Ivanova, M. I., Sievers, S. A., Apostol, M. I., Thompson, M. J., Balbirnie, M., Wiltzius, J. J. W., McFarlane, H. T., Madsen, A. O., Riekel, C., and Eisenberg, D. (2007) Atomic structures of amyloid cross-beta spines reveal varied steric zippers. *Nature* **447**, 453–457.

Scheibel, T., Parthasarathy, R., Sawicki, G., Lin, X. M., Jaeger, H., and Lindquist, S. L. (2003) Conducting nanowires built by controlled self-assembly of amyloid fibers and selective metal deposition. *Proc. Natl. Acad. Sci. USA* **100**, 4527–4532.

Schinazi, R. F., Sijbesma, R., Srdanov, G., Hill, C. L., and Wudl, F. (1993) Synthesis and virucidal activity of a water-soluble, configurationally stable, derivatized C60 fullerene. *Antimicrob. Agents Chemother.* **37**, 1707–1710.

Schneider, J. P., Pochan, D. J., Ozbas, B., Rajagopal, K., Pakstis, L., and Kretsinger, J. (2002) Responsive hydrogels from the intramolecular folding and self-assembly of a designed peptide. *J. Am. Chem. Soc.* **124**, 15030–15037.

Schnorr, J. M. and Swager, T. M. (2011) Emerging applications of carbon nanotubes. *Chem. Mater.* **23**, 646–657.

Schuster, B., Gyorvary, E., Pum, D., and Sleytr, U. B. (2005) Nanotechnology with S-layer proteins. *Methods Mol. Biol.* **300**, 101–123.

Seeman, N. C. (1990) *De novo* design of sequences for nucleic acid structural engineering. *J. Biomol. Struct. Dyn.* **8**, 573–581.

Seeman, N. C. (2005) Structural DNA nanotechnology: An overview. *Methods Mol. Biol.* **303**, 143–166.

Seeman, N. C. (2010) Structural DNA nanotechnology: Growing along with nano letters. *Nano Lett.* **10**, 1971–1978.

Seil, J. T. and Webster, T. J. (2010) Electrically active nanomaterials as improved neural tissue regeneration scaffolds. *Wiley Interdiscip. Rev. Nanomed. Nanobiotechnol.* **2**, 635–647.

Sherman, W. B. and Seeman, N. C. (2006) Design of minimally strained nucleic acid nanotubes. *Biophys. J.* **90**, 4546–4557.

Shim, J., Bersano-Begey, T. F., Zhu, X., Tkaczyk, A. H., Linderman, J. J., and Takayama, S. (2003) Micro- and nanotechnologies for studying cellular function. *Curr. Top. Med. Chem.* **3**, 687–703.

Shimizu, K., Cha, J., Stucky, G. D., and Morse, D. E. (1998) Silicatein alpha: Cathepsin L-like protein in sponge biosilica. *Proc. Natl. Acad. Sci. USA* **95**, 6234–6238.

Shklovsky, J., Beker, P., Amdursky, N., Gazit, E., and Rosenman, G. (2010) Bioinspired peptide nanotubes: Deposition technology and physical properties. *Mat. Sci. Eng. B-Solid* **169**, 62–66.

Silva, G. A., Czeisler, C., Niece, K. L., Beniash, E., Harrington, D. A., Kessler, J. A., and Stupp, S. I. (2004) Selective differentiation of neural progenitor cells by high-epitope density nanofibers. *Science* **303**, 1352–1355.

Smith, A. M. and Scheibel, T. (2010) Functional amyloids used by organisms: A lesson in controlling assembly. *Macromol. Chem. Physic.* **211**, 127–135.

Smith, K. H., Tejeda-Montes, E., Poch, M., and Mata, A. (2011) Integrating top-down and self-assembly in the fabrication of peptide and protein-based biomedical materials. *Chem. Soc. Rev.* **40**, 4563–4577.

Song, Y. J., Challa, S. R., Medforth, C. J., Qiu, Y., Watt, R. K., Pena, D., Miller, J. E., van Swol, F., and Shelnutt, J. A. (2004) Synthesis of peptide-nanotube platinum-nanoparticle composites. *Chem. Commun.* **9**, 1044–1045.

Spiess, K., Lammel, A., and Scheibel, T. (2010) Recombinant spider silk proteins for applications in biomaterials. *Macromol. Biosci.* **10**, 998–1007.

Stevens, M. M. and Mecklenburg, G. (2012) Bio-inspired materials for biosensing and tissue engineering. *Polym. Int.* **61**, 680–685.

Sundar, V. C., Yablon, A. D., Grazul, J. L., Ilan, M., and Aizenberg, J. (2003) Fibre-optical features of a glass sponge. *Nature* **424**, 899–900.

Tahir, M. N., Theato, P., Muller, W. E. G., Schroder, H. C., Borejko, A., Faiss, S., Janshoff, A., Huth, J., and Tremel, W. (2005) Formation of layered titania and zirconia catalysed by surface-bound silicatein. *Chem. Commun.* **44**, 5533–5535.

Tamerler, C., Khatayevich, D., Gungormus, M., Kacar, T., Oren, E. E., Hnilova, M., and Sarikaya, M. (2010) Molecular Biomimetics: GEPI-based biological routes to technology. *Biopolymers* **94**, 78–94.

Taniguchi, N. (1974) On the basic concept of 'nanotechnology'. *Proc. Intl. Conf. Prod. Eng. Tokyo, Part II,* Japan Society of Precision Engineering.

Tenidis, K., Waldner, M., Bernhagen, J., Fischle, W., Bergmann, M., Weber, M., Merkle, M. L., Voelter, W., Brunner, H., and Kapurniotu, A. (2000) Identification of a penta- and hexapeptide of islet amyloid polypeptide (IAPP) with amyloidogenic and cytotoxic properties. *J. Mol. Biol.* **295**, 1055–1071.

Tenne, R. (2002) Inorganic nanotubes and fullerene-like materials. *Chemistry* **8**, 5296–5304.

Tenne, R. (2006) Inorganic nanotubes and fullerene-like nanoparticles. *Nat. Nanotechnol.* **1**, 103–111.

Tenne, R. and Rao, C. N. (2004) Inorganic nanotubes. *Philos. Transact. A. Math. Phys. Eng. Sci.* **362**, 2099–2125.

True, H. L., Berlin, I., and Lindquist, S. L. (2004) Epigenetic regulation of translation reveals hidden genetic variation to produce complex traits. *Nature* **431**, 184–187.

Valery, C., Paternostre, M., Robert, B., Gulik-Krzywicki, T., Narayanan, T., Dedieu, J. C., Keller, G., Torres, M. L., Cherif-Cheikh, R., Calvo, P., and Artzner, F. (2003) Biomimetic organization: Octapeptide self-assembly into nanotubes of viral capsid-like dimension. *Proc. Natl. Acad. Sci. USA* **100**, 10258–10262.

Valery, C., Artzner, F., and Paternostre, M. (2011) Peptide nanotubes: Molecular organisations, self-assembly mechanisms and applications. *Soft Matter*, **7**, 9583–9594.

Vassanelli S., Mahmud M., Girardi S., and Maschietto M. (2012) On the way to large-scale and high-resolution brain-chip interfacing. *Cognitive Computation* **4**, 71–81.

Vauthey, S., Santoso, S., Gong, H., Watson, N., and Zhang, S. (2002) Molecular self-assembly of surfactant-like peptides to form nanotubes and nanovesicles. *Proc. Natl. Acad. Sci. USA* **99**, 5355–5360.

Venkatesan, B. M. and Bashir, R. (2011) Nanopore sensors for nucleic acid analysis. *Nat. Nanotechnol.* **6**, 615–624.

Wagner, D. E., Phillips, C. L., Ali, W. M., Nybakken, G. E., Crawford, E. D., Schwab, A. D., Smith, W. F., and Fairman, R. (2005) Toward the development of peptide nanofilaments and nanoropes as smart materials. *Proc. Natl. Acad. Sci. USA* **102**, 12656–12661.

Walter, P., Welcomme, E., Hallegot, P., Zaluzec, N. J., Deeb, C., Castaing, J., Veyssiere, P., Breniaux, R., Leveque, J. L., and Tsoucaris, G. (2006) Early use of PbS nanotechnology for an ancient hair dyeing formula. *Nano Lett.* **6**, 2215–2219.

Wang, T., Schiffels, D., Cuesta, S. M., Fygenson, D. K., and Seeman, N. C. (2012) Design and characterization of 1d nanotubes and 2d periodic arrays self-assembled from DNA multi-helix bundles. *J. Am. Chem. Soc.* **134**, 1606–1616.

Wang, W. U., Chen, C., Lin, K. H., Fang, Y., and Lieber, C. M. (2005) Label-free detection of small-molecule-protein interactions by using nanowire nanosensors. *Proc. Natl. Acad. Sci. USA* **102**, 3208–3212.

Wang, Y. C. and Ho, C. C. (2004) Micropatterning of proteins and mammalian cells on biomaterials. *FASEB J.* **18**, 525–527.

Weiner, S., Sagi, I., and Addadi, L. (2005) Structural biology. Choosing the crystallization path less traveled. *Science* **309**, 1027–1028.

Weisman, S., Okada, S., Mudie, S. T., Huson, M. G., Trueman, H. E., Sriskantha, A., Haritos, V. S., and Sutherland, T. D. (2009) Fifty years later: The sequence, structure and function of lacewing cross-beta silk. *J. Struct. Biol.* **168**, 467–475.

Whitesides, G. M., Mathias, J. P., and Seto, C. T. (1991) Molecular self-assembly and nanochemistry: A chemical strategy for the synthesis of nanostructures. *Science* **254**, 1312–1319.

Whitesides, G. M., Ostuni, E., Takayama, S., Jiang, X., and Ingber, D. E. (2001) Soft lithography in biology and biochemistry. *Annu. Rev. Biomed. Eng.* **3**, 335–373.

Wilchek, M. and Bayer, E. A. (1990) Introduction to avidin-biotin technology. *Methods Enzymol.* **184**, 5–13.

Woolfson, D. N. (2010) Building fibrous biomaterials from alpha-helical and collagen-like coiled-coil peptides. *Biopolymers* **94**, 118–127.

Wu, E. C., Zhang, S. G., and Hauser, C. A. E. (2012) Self-assembling peptides as cell-interactive scaffolds. *Adv. Funct. Mater.* **22**, 456–468.

Wu, H., Wheeler, A., Zare, R. N. (2004) Chemical cytometry on a picoliter-scale integrated microfluidic chip. *Proc. Natl. Acad. Sci. USA* **101**, 12809–12813.

Yager, P. and Schoen, P. E. (1984) Formation of tubules by a polymerizable surfactant. *Mol. Cryst. Liq. Cryst.* **106**, 371–381.

Yamada, K., Ihara, H., Ide, T., Fukumoto, T., and Hirayama, C. (1984) Formation of helical super structure from single-walled bilayers by amphiphiles with oligo-L-glutamic acid-head group. *Chem. Lett.* **1984**, 1713–1716.

Yemini, M., Reches, M., Gazit, E., and Rishpon, J. (2005a) Peptide nanotube-modified electrodes for enzyme-biosensors applications. *Anal. Chem.* **77**, 5155–5159.

Yemini, M., Reches, M., Rishpon, J., and Gazit, E. (2005b) Novel electrochemical biosensing platform using self-assembled peptide nanotubes. *Nano Lett.* **5**, 183–186.

Zhang, S. (2003) Fabrication of novel biomaterials through molecular self-assembly. *Nat. Biotechnol.* **21**, 1171–1178.

Zhao, C. X., Yu, L., and Middelberg, A. P. J. (2012) Design of low-charge peptide sequences for high-yield formation of titania nanoparticles. *RSC Advances* **2**, 1292–1295.

Zheng, G., Patolsky, F., Cui, Y., Wang, W. U., and Lieber, C. M. (2005) Multiplexed electrical detection of cancer markers with nanowire sensor arrays. *Nat. Biotechnol.* **23**, 1294–1301.

Zimenkov, Y., Conticello, V. P., Guo, L., and Thiyagarajan, P. (2004) Rational design of a nanoscale helical scaffold derived from self-assembly of a dimeric coiled coil motif. *Tetrahedron* **60**, 7237–7246.

Index